PRAISE FOR *THE INFLU*
TRAUMA

"*From beginning to end,* The Influence of Psychological Trauma in Nursing *is a remarkable contribution to the discipline and practice of nursing. The text brings together insights gained from research, theory, and practice to explain how psychological trauma—both the nurse's and the patient's—is experienced and outlines the paths to recovery and healing. Throughout the book there are real-life stories to illustrate the major concepts and invitations to reflect on one's own experiences and practices. Most notably, this book is true to the fundamental values and purposes of nursing, explaining how nursing theory and nursing's patterns of knowing provide ways to organize competent, trauma-informed nursing care. This book should be required for every nursing student at every educational level (including continuing education). It will revolutionize how nurses think, how they engage with their own experience and with one another, and ultimately, how nursing is practiced.*"

–Peggy L. Chinn, PhD, RN, FAAN
Professor Emerita, University of Connecticut
Editor, *Advances in Nursing Science*

"*Finally! A book that explains psychological trauma in an understandable fashion, based on science. The most pressing public health problems in the US today, addictions and suicide, usually have trauma precursors. Yet nursing education has not provided a coherent path to understanding trauma's basic concepts. Authors Foli and Thompson have written a book that each nursing school should integrate into its curricula, both undergraduate and graduate. By doing so, RNs will understand that the phenomena they encounter in everyday practice are rooted in psychological trauma and will be equipped to implement evidence-based treatments for remediation.*"

–Teena M. McGuinness, PhD, CRNP, FAANP, FAAN
Professor, University of Alabama at Birmingham School of Nursing

"*Trauma is all around us. This text is essential reading for our times, preparing nurses to address ancestral and patient trauma, as well as their own trauma. Through stories, reflections, conceptual models, nursing theories, and research, this book provides the latest evidence on how to unveil and heal from trauma during the formative years of nursing education to engage in professional nursing praxis from a place of self-awareness with wisdom, courage, and compassion.*"

–Sara Horton-Deutsch, PhD, RN, PMHCNS, FAAN, ANEF, Caritas Coach
Professor, University of San Francisco School of Nursing and Health Professions

"This text is a much-needed compilation of the literature on trauma and nursing. The authors have thoughtfully organized each chapter with trauma-informed reflections and excellent case examples. All nurses and nursing students should read this book to understand the pervasive effect of trauma on health and learning and the impact of trauma on nurses as caregivers. As an academic, I especially appreciated the application of trauma-informed content to the AACN Essentials of Baccalaureate Education for Professional Nursing Practice. The quality of this book is outstanding, with the latest research on trauma rendered in reader-friendly prose."

–Kathleen Wheeler, PhD, PMHNP-BC, APRN, FAAN
Professor, Fairfield University Egan School of Nursing and Health Studies

"Trauma, whether the big T (loss of a family member) or the little t (a friend moves away), affects the body's systems and the brain's architecture. This book provides the knowledge and skills to address self and patient symptoms precipitated by trauma. The authors engagingly describe the causes of trauma and the constructive ways that nurses can respond, based on research evidence, solid experience, and insightful wisdom. A true companion to promote a rewarding practice."

–Genevieve E. Chandler, PhD, RN, Resilience Expert
Associate Professor, University of Massachusetts Amherst

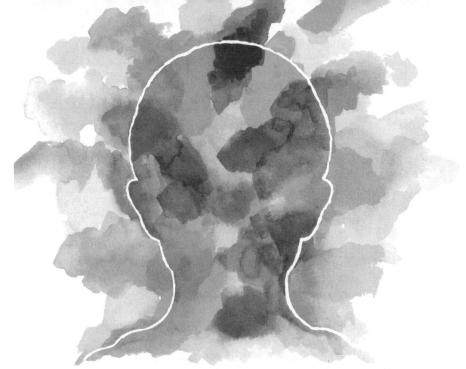

The Influence of
Psychological
Trauma
in Nursing

Karen J. Foli, PhD, RN, FAAN
John R. Thompson, MD

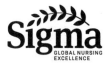

Sigma
GLOBAL NURSING
EXCELLENCE

The Sigma Theta Tau International Honor Society of Nursing (Sigma) is a nonprofit organization whose mission is advancing world health and celebrating nursing excellence in scholarship, leadership, and service. Founded in 1922, Sigma has more than 135,000 active members in over 90 countries and territories. Members include practicing nurses, instructors, researchers, policymakers, entrepreneurs, and others. Sigma's more than 530 chapters are located at more than 700 institutions of higher education throughout Armenia, Australia, Botswana, Brazil, Canada, Colombia, England, Ghana, Hong Kong, Ireland, Japan, Jordan, Kenya, Lebanon, Malawi, Mexico, the Netherlands, Nigeria, Pakistan, Philippines, Portugal, Puerto Rico, Singapore, South Africa, South Korea, Swaziland, Sweden, Taiwan, Tanzania, Thailand, the United States, and Wales. Learn more at www.sigmanursing.org.

Sigma Theta Tau International
550 West North Street
Indianapolis, IN, USA 46202

To order additional books, buy in bulk, or order for corporate use, contact Sigma Marketplace at 888.654.4968 (US and Canada) or +1.317.634.8171 (outside US and Canada).

To request a review copy for course adoption or for more information about the ancillary Instructor's Guide and Student Workbook, email solutions@sigmamarketplace.org or call 888.654.4968 (US and Canada) or +1.317.634.8171 (outside US and Canada).

To request author information, or for speaker or other media requests, contact Sigma Marketing at 888.634.7575 (US and Canada) or +1.317.634.8171 (outside US and Canada).

ISBN:	9781945157981
EPUB ISBN:	9781945157998
PDF ISBN:	9781948057004
MOBI ISBN:	9781948057011

Library of Congress Cataloging-in-Publication data

Names: Foli, Karen J., author. | Thompson, John R., M.D., author.
Title: The influence of psychological trauma in nursing / Karen J. Foli, John R. Thompson.
Description: Indianapolis, IN : Sigma Theta Tau International, [2019]
Identifiers: LCCN 2019013692 (print) | LCCN 2019014694 (ebook) | ISBN 9781945157998 (epub) | ISBN 9781948057004 (pdf) | ISBN 9781948057011 (mobi) | ISBN 9781945157981 (print) | ISBN 9781948057011 (mobi)
Subjects: | MESH: Psychological Trauma | Nurse-Patient Relations | Nursing Care--methods | Nurses Instruction
Classification: LCC RC552.T7 (ebook) | LCC RC552.T7 (print) | NLM WM 172.5 | DDC 616.85/210231--dc23

First Printing, 2019

Publisher: Dustin Sullivan	**Managing Editor:** Carla Hall
Acquisitions Editor: Emily Hatch	**Development and Project Editor:** Rebecca Senninger
Publications Specialist: Todd Lothery	
Cover Designer: Rebecca Batchelor	**Copy Editor:** Gill Editorial Services
Interior Design/Page Layout: Rebecca Batchelor	**Proofreader:** Todd Lothery
	Indexer: Joy Dean Lee

Instructuor's Guide and Student Workbook are available for this textbook. Contact solutions@sigmamarketplace or call 888.654.4968 (US and Canada) or +1.317.634.8171 (outside US and Canada) for more information.

DEDICATIONS

This book is dedicated to nurses who seek healing
from trauma within themselves and who seek healing for others.

And to Mark Conway, MD, our beloved family member,
whose gentle spirit and quiet strength
helped us understand true compassion and love.

ACKNOWLEDGMENTS

The goal of any work is to ensure that the aim and audience are always kept in the center of the authors' efforts. Our aim—to increase insight into personal trauma and build trauma awareness and resilience in new nurses—was always in the forefront of our energies. As we sought to secure a home for this book, we believed this book was needed and would ultimately improve the quality of nurses' lives and enhance patient-centered care.

Personally, we want to extend our thanks to family and friends. To our children, Ben, Peter, and Annie: You give us purpose in our lives and grace us with your love. The support from our extended family is so appreciated: Leanne and Bill Malloy, Katie Malloy, Margaret Conway, Jeff Conway, Dave and Tana Conway, and Adele Foli. To our beloved family members who recently left us, Reno Foli and Mark Conway, you are very much missed and remembered with love. Others who have impacted our lives and cheered us on include Patricia Moisan-Thomas, Melanie Braswell, Karen Sanders, Janet Thorlton, Becky Walters, Kristen Kirby, Cindy Bozich-Keith, and Rhonda Moravec. Thank you all for your support.

A big thank you to Geraldine Pearson for introducing this work to readers. She skillfully situates our message in a historical, professional, and autobiographical manner. Her generous spirit and expertise are sincerely noted and appreciated.

We are grateful to Sigma and its publishing staff. To Emily Hatch, thank you for our first meeting during which you advised Karen to think more broadly in nursing education, while focusing the work. To Carla Hall, for encouragement, great communication throughout the process, and assisting with book graphics and permissions. To Dustin Sullivan, who supported and celebrated with us as we completed this book. And finally, to the Sigma publishing committee, who requested companion books so that students could apply trauma-informed nursing care through simulations. In summary, thank you for believing in this book.

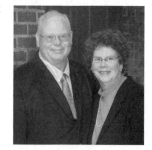

ABOUT THE AUTHORS

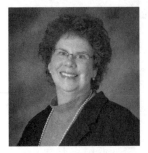 **Karen J. Foli, PhD, RN, FAAN,** received her associate's and bachelor's degrees from Indiana State University and her master's degree, with an emphasis in nursing administration, from Indiana University School of Nursing, Indianapolis. Dr. Foli received her PhD in communications from the University of Illinois, Urbana–Champaign. She is an Associate Professor and the Director of the PhD in Nursing Program at Purdue University School of Nursing, West Lafayette, Indiana.

Foli is a fellow in the American Academy of Nursing (AAN) in recognition for her work with nontraditional families, such as adoption and kinship families. She is a member of the Child, Adolescent, and Family Expert Panel through the AAN. She has forwarded a mid-range theory of parental postadoption depression and has tested this theory in empirical studies. Her research is bound together to alleviate the suffering of psychological trauma. She is currently examining the role of psychological trauma in substance use in registered nurses.

A recipient of numerous teaching awards, including the Charles B. Murphy Outstanding Undergraduate Teaching Award from Purdue University, the highest award bestowed for undergraduate teaching at the university, Foli takes pride in being a nurse educator. In 2018, she was one of 45 faculty members who were inducted into the Purdue University Book of Great Teachers, signifying excellence in teaching. She also received the Sigma Theta Tau International Honor Society of Nursing Delta Omicron Chapter Award for Outstanding Mentoring in 2017. Preparing nurse scientists is also an important part of Foli's professional work. As the director of the PhD in Nursing Program, she encourages and guides students and faculty in preparing nurses who will continue to explore and build upon the science of nursing.

Foli's lifelong love of writing has produced works in a wide range of formats and genres, including memoir, regulatory writing in the pharmaceutical industry, scholarly writing of empirical studies, and mystery short stories. She is author or coauthor of four well-received health-related books. One of these, *Nursing Care of Adoption and Kinship Families: A Clinical Guide for Advanced Practice Nurses* (2017, Springer), received the American Psychiatric Nurses Association (APNA) Award for Media in 2018. This award "recognizes APNA members who have demonstrated excellence in producing media related to psychiatric-mental health nursing."

A special passion of Foli's work is advancing the conceptualization of nursing and the "work" of nurses. The elusive definition of nursing motivates her efforts to forward a way to value and communicate what nurses do in practice, in education, in policy, and in research. She has partnered with many graduate students and coauthored several papers that define important concepts surrounding nursing care.

Her appreciation for nurses and the profession of nursing is unique in that her career path veered away from the profession for a time and carried her into professional writing, teaching business communications in a Big Ten business school, and writing global experimental research protocols for a large pharmaceutical company. When she returned to the world of nursing, Foli realized how much society needs the special comfort, caring, and compassion offered by nurses. Her deep appreciation for what nurses experience motivated her to write this book to prepare students and those new to the field to become stronger and more resilient as they process and encounter patients in crises and in need of trauma-informed care.

Foli and her coauthor, John R. Thompson, have been married for almost three decades and have three adult children. Avid dog lovers, they have always been owners of at least three dogs, many times taking in strays and "dumped" animals who became loved members of their family.

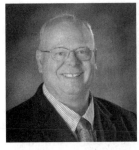

John R. Thompson, MD, has practiced as a physician in the specialty area of psychiatry for the past 30 years. He completed his residency in general psychiatry and a fellowship in child/adolescent psychiatry in the Department of Psychiatry at Indiana University. Since Thompson's fellowship, he has worked with a variety of populations, including children, adolescents, young adults, and adults, including addiction psychiatry. He has practiced in multiple healthcare contexts: acute care/inpatient care, intensive outpatient, community mental health, consult-liaison, veterans' mental health, and forensic psychiatry. Along with Karen Foli, he is coauthor of *The Post-Adoption Blues: Overcoming the Unforeseen Challenges of Adoption* (Rodale, 2004).

Currently, he practices psychiatric medicine for Purdue University's Counseling and Psychological Services, West Lafayette, Indiana. In this position, Thompson evaluates and manages the psychiatric needs of students enrolled in higher education. Common issues include depression, anxiety, substance use, personality disorders, attention deficit disorder, and healing from trauma.

Thompson is also a cancer survivor; thus, his insights into trauma are both personal and professional. In his medical practice, he assesses and counsels young adults who are processing and recovering from trauma. Thompson approaches the individual in a trauma-informed, holistic way. He strives to promote a feeling of safety and allows the individual to share past experiences as the relationship is built and trust evolves. He believes in "de-prescribing" medications—removing those agents that create addictions, lack a therapeutic rationale, or are interacting with other agents in nontherapeutic ways. Taking time to review past medical records, Thompson pieces together past traumas, dual diagnoses, and concurrent medical conditions that, when revealed, contribute to optimal care. Recognizing that healthcare disparities and social determinants of health result in individuals struggling to secure resources in filling prescriptions and in the wider community, he searches for affordable healthcare and orders appropriate referrals to provide for a continuum of care.

Growing up in the Rocky Mountains of Colorado, Thompson enjoys nature and being outdoors. His spirit is recharged upon seeing growth both in his plants and trees, and more importantly, in people. Being part of students' success, seeing them achieve their career goals as they develop as young adults, motivates Thompson to continue to offer each individual his best efforts as a medical provider.

TABLE OF CONTENTS

1 UNDERSTANDING PSYCHOLOGICAL TRAUMA 1

2 TRAUMA AND BECOMING A NURSE 31

FOREWORD

The Influence of Psychological Trauma in Nursing, by Karen J. Foli and
John R. Thompson, is an outstanding book and an essential read for all
nurses, regardless of specialty, practice site, or education level. While
the book is particularly applicable to psychiatric nurses, it is useful to all
nurses regardless of setting. Though not all nurses come to the profession
with past trauma, few nurses practice without experiencing some trauma
or stress as they provide care. As Foli and Thompson so eloquently note,
these experiences are part of the caring role of nursing, with its emphasis
on humanistic, attentive, and intentional practice. Trauma is a hazard of
providing good nursing care.

As I read the introduction to this book, I was transported back to my
years as a nursing student who was drawn early on to psychiatric nursing, curious about what had created the human struggles I already saw
across the life span. In 1972 there was little mention of trauma as the
root cause of so many physical and mental health problems I saw in my
patients. These included the elder veteran on the medical-surgical unit at
a Veteran's Administration hospital, with pancreatitis and alcoholism and
numerous medals for heroism; the drama of my first obstetrical patient,
barely 12 years old and pregnant from sexual abuse; and the 7-year-old boy
in a state-run group home for foster children. I volunteered in that group
home as a sophomore in nursing school at the recommendation of my
faculty advisor, who saw my leanings toward child psychiatric nursing. It
was a pivotal career moment, as I got to observe and work with a houseful
of children who had experienced so much stress in their young lives. The
child assigned to me for play was a boy who quickly latched on to me with
an intensity and neediness that baffled and frightened me. As I concluded
that placement, I remember him tearfully begging me to take him to my
house so I could be his mother. I was 19 years old.

My point in this self-revelation is to emphasize that 40 years ago
in nursing, there was little discussion of trauma as the root of so many
healthcare issues encountered by nurses. As I went to graduate school
and on to a job in a federally funded community clinic, I saw many foster
children who were dealing with the loss of family, the trauma of placement, and the early experiences that had initially put them into foster care.

I didn't have an anchor to understand what they were presenting to me or the skills to effectively intervene. This continued into a faculty position, followed by a clinical nurse specialist role in a state psychiatric hospital for children. The trauma was described but not named as a specific event with an outcome. The staff watched it, lived it, and tried to intervene. I often wondered what effect this environment had on the people around me, the nurses and childcare workers. Most of their energy went toward managing these incredibly damaged children and their symptoms. I saw a lot of compassion fatigue during that time.

After I got my PhD in nursing, I took a faculty position in a medical school where my office was next to a trauma researcher. He focused almost entirely on intervention models with clients and built a successful academic career around this. As the only nurse in the department, I often wondered how nurses, who I realized by then were different in the ways they approached and understood the people they worked with, dealt personally with these issues. So many of the nurses I knew (including me) had their own trauma history that they worked on and had to partially resolve to do the work. While I realized that all clinicians had to know the transference and countertransference issues influencing their work, I thought nurses were specifically vulnerable to the stress of working with traumatized individuals. And honestly, weren't all the people we saw directly or indirectly suffering from the effects of some sort of trauma?

This book is a beautifully nuanced, thorough description of the definitions of trauma, the theoretical underpinnings, and the nursing theory that defines assessment and interventions. It is liberally sprinkled with carefully crafted case studies and examples. It speaks volumes to nurses who are practicing in many settings with patients, other nurses, and students.

I am happy to say that there is currently a different level of attention to the issues of trauma that influence our practice and care as psychiatric nurses. I now do a thorough trauma assessment on every child and adolescent presenting for outpatient care in my practice. I have trauma treatment resources readily available, and I can now put a name to the reactions I repeatedly see in parents and children that have roots in trauma.

In an ideal world, trauma would not occur, but this, of course, is unrealistic. We are fortunate to have books like this one that provide the specific support nurses need beyond the usual descriptors of trauma and trauma treatment. Kudos to these authors for this important work!

–Geraldine S. Pearson, PhD, PMH-CNS, APRN, FAAN
Editor-in-Chief, *Journal of the American Psychiatric Nurses Association*
Associate Professor–retired, UConn School of Medicine
Co-Chairperson, Committee on Publication Ethics (COPE)

INTRODUCTION

"You must not lose faith in humanity. Humanity is an ocean; if a few
drops of the ocean are dirty, the ocean does not become dirty."
—Mahatma Gandhi

Welcome! In this book, you'll find a confluence of words surrounding the concept of "psychological trauma." Some of these words will apply directly to you and your image of who and what you are. Some of these words will apply to you in the context of nursing and the act of rendering care to others. The beginning quote by Mahatma Gandhi reflects that trauma is a two-party system: Someone is the receiver of trauma, and another is the giver of trauma—intentional or unintentional. Gandhi's words remind us, however, to take a broader view in that the world is bigger than those who are responsible for trauma in others.

We begin with a story told by Karen:

She stumbled into my office, a petite young woman with thick, dark, long hair. I looked up, distracted by a manuscript I was drafting. In the middle of earning tenure at a university, I was a "poster child" for today's nursing faculty: middle-aged (and then some), yet driven to produce in the "three-legged stool" of academia: discovery, teaching, and engagement. She sat across from my desk in a lopsided way and calmly told me that because she was in one of my courses, I ought to know: "I was raped over the weekend."

As a nurse, I've seen babies born and individuals take their last breaths, but for a few seconds, I could only stare at this young woman. People who go to school to become nurses change. It is not just a major in school; the "nurse" is swallowed inside us and becomes part of who we become as people. I paused, blinked, and the nurse stepped up. The questions spilled into one another: "Are you all right?" "Have you reported this?" "Whom did you report this to?" Then I stopped and looked into her face. Her features became paralyzed as she stared at me.

Those weren't the questions she needed right now. She needed me to reach out to her and with her, to acknowledge the hurt and pain, and to offer acceptance and support. After this pause, we actually communicated.

I listened, and I saw and felt her tears. She led and I followed. But I also knew that I wasn't going to let her out of my office without connecting her to services. Looking back, her case was straightforward: The appropriate people (legal, medical for her physical injuries, and academic) had been notified. She thought she was done, but I knew her survivorship and healing would be molded in the next few days, and then the next few months, and onward after that.

She told me she was fine. It was over. She wanted to go on with her life. I wanted that too but knew that work—very hard work—needed to be done. Together, we walked a few blocks to the on-campus crisis center located in the Psychological Sciences department. I waited in the room with her and helped her fill out the intake form. After what seemed like hours but was only a few minutes, she was called back to see the on-call therapist. After she had left, I stared at the pictures on the wall, the posters that advertised various student services, and the outdated magazines on the side table beside me. I thought of her parents. I had two boys and a little girl. I wondered what I would feel if it were my child. I thought of the young man who had hurt her. I wondered about his parents and whether they knew. I wondered about loss and sadness at such a young age. I thought about the media and how people were objectified. I thought about all this as the hard wood of the chair pressed up against my back. I thought about psychological trauma.

Before leaving my office, I had galvanized my backup and resources: the director of the student's program. After receiving my message that I needed to speak with her, she stepped out of a meeting and arrived at the counseling office as soon as she could. Slightly out of breath, she sat down next to me. About the same age as I am, Julia[1] was one of those nurses you couldn't help but admire. She was the whole "package" as a nurse: decades of clinical experience, pragmatic, honestly straightforward with feedback, and brilliant. We sat there in the Psychological Services clinic, and I communicated to her what had happened. There was something about the two of us sitting there in those hard wooden chairs. We were two nurses, two women, who had experienced life in good and bad ways, and we shared our sadness in silence. And we waited for this student, whom we cared very much about, to emerge from her first session.

---

[1]*My colleague's name has been changed to further protect the student's identity.*

Over the ensuing weeks, Julia and I put together a plan to support our student. One day during our regular meetings, I watched as Julia pulled some papers out of the copy machine. She reached for a marker and began writing on the top sheet.

"What are you doing?" I asked.

She smiled, and I watched as Julia flipped the page to show me. It was a calendar that extended to the end of the school year, with X's showing the days that had passed.

"This way, she'll know there's an end in sight." Julia turned back to the sheet, and her smile was replaced by a look of sorrow.

Julia and I became closer as we supported the student, who felt so unsafe and unsure. Her go-to support system of peers had abandoned her, taking sides over the assault, trying to make sense of it by assigning blame. We knew her class schedule and ensured she walked with someone to and from each class. Julia took the majority of the escorted trips, and gradually, the student felt more at ease. Many times, I saw Julia walking across campus so that at the end of her class, the student had someone present with her to provide that feeling of safety as she went to the next classroom. We became new social connections for her, and she forged ahead with the goal of finishing the program. Finally, after a few weeks, graduation arrived.

After the school's recognition ceremony, which included a pinning ceremony and the Nightingale Pledge being recited, parents and students approached faculty and asked for photos and received handshakes of congratulations. Emerging from the crowd, I saw her approaching me with her mom—the same dark hair—and her father. Their faces, their smiles, their steps toward me, each a showcase of joy and hurt, as if a wound in each of them had yet to heal and the presence on campus had carved a fresh layer of pain. They greeted me. I saw each of their features in their daughter and then, a gift bag and a card were offered to me. Words of gratitude were spoken, "We can't thank you enough for what you did for our daughter." I murmured how brave she was and how I knew the future would be bright and fresh. She had secured a wonderful professional opportunity out of state.

I will always remember this student—her experiences, her courage, and my friend Julia's kindness and trauma-informed support. The student taught me about resiliency, healing, compassion, and the power of being connected to other human beings. These are important in the transition from victim to survivor. She taught me about educating students whose lives had been affected by trauma. The purpose of this book is for individuals who are becoming nurses to begin to recognize past traumas in their lives—how these experiences may affect behaviors and perceptions of others, as well as the trauma experienced by those they render care to.

YOUR TRAUMA "SCRIPT"

Perhaps you recognize yourself or someone you know in the story Karen just shared. If not the specific injury, the student's experiences after a traumatic event may have reminded you, become a trigger, of an event in your life. This event might have occurred in your past, in childhood for example, or more recently. Diagnoses such as attention deficit disorder and learning disabilities can carry with them labels such as "lazy," "stupid," and "broken." Overcoming an initial traumatic event, such as physical and emotional injuries in a car accident, can precipitate another trauma, such as the loss of function. Sometimes, we may not consciously recognize when trauma has occurred until later when we've had time to reflect and process it—or be reminded of it through a real-time event.

Now you're in nursing school and may be faced with additional forms of trauma related to offering comfort to others in times of crisis and extreme vulnerability. In life, we experience many universal emotions, including love, joy, and hope. We are compelled to add that, for many of us, experiencing trauma is also a common thread. Nurses are unique creatures who listen to, empathize with, and at times, grieve with individuals they render care to. It is important to understand your "trauma script" as you read these pages because you take on many roles in society, and trauma touches each of us in different ways.

You have a cultural and historical context that brings with it experiences, both good and bad, that have shaped who you are. You or a family member/friend may have experienced significant trauma. Nursing as a profession has yet to achieve gender balance, and therefore, as women, we have experienced our own trauma or been caregivers to those who have.

Yet, as men increasingly join the nursing workforce, they also bring with them stories of trauma, such as sexual harassment, from both patients and managers. Sons and daughters, partners, mothers, and fathers—we care for them, literally and figuratively. Trauma affects not only the person who has experienced it but also those who are indirectly involved. You may be part of this second layer of trauma. In other words, no one is without some exposure to psychological trauma. The overall goal of this book is twofold: to help you recognize trauma (in yourself and others) and to learn ways of recovering from trauma so that you can heal and bring holistic healing to others.

AIMS OF THIS BOOK

We take this opportunity to clarify that this is not a "self-help" book. It is also not a substitute for a therapeutic relationship with a mental health provider or a proxy for support from family and friends. However, this text is an important first step in becoming aware of how trauma may have influenced you as an individual and/or those around you, including peers and family. We discuss a viewpoint that includes the psychological implications of trauma's effects, why people who have been traumatized act in the ways they do, and how to intervene in smart, informed ways as you render care as a nurse. Specifically, our goals are:

To expand your understanding of what psychological trauma is and what types of trauma exist in society today. Although nurses are caring professionals with unique knowledge and skills, we also recognize that trauma invades internal and external environments. This book offers a primer on conceptualizing psychological trauma and understanding the common forms of trauma in society. It is meant to provide a foundation of knowledge in this area so that you can move forward as a caregiver in a "trauma-informed" way. Being trauma-informed means that you see individuals' behaviors through the lens of how trauma impacts an individual. Their behaviors may appear to be odd, difficult, hostile, or even aggressive. Internally, they may be struggling with a need to feel safe, low self-esteem, anxiety, sadness, loneliness, or depression. This book describes the "why" behind how people who have experienced trauma may feel and act.

To increase your personal insight into your past, present, and potential future experiences that may be traumatic. Our trauma scripts are with us, similar to a physical feature that may change with time but is in some form a part of us. It is not that we want to be reminded of past trauma; instead, often we suppress, ignore, minimize, or intellectualize our past hurts and harms. By reading this book, you may begin to appreciate what has happened in your life and brought you to this point of becoming a nurse, and you may make sense of the whispers of past traumas. We describe some of the particular ways that nurses are vulnerable to both physical and psychological trauma. We know that trauma can instill a fear of the future, one's prediction that outcomes will always be negative. Thus, stress increases. But the right amount of stress can serve to motivate us, provide a sharper focus. It is finding that balance between motivating stress and toxic stress that we want to achieve. Despite the fact that we are a caring and trustworthy group of professionals, nurses continue to be targets of peer and supervisor bullying and targets of violence in the workplace. This brings us to another theme that we want to weave into our book.

To build a resilient workforce who is prepared to process and heal from trauma and help others heal. The duality of personal and patient-focused trauma is real, and as nurses, the more centered we feel, the more we can offer to our patients. It is important to understand how certain populations may be more vulnerable to psychological trauma: those involved with natural disasters or war-time activities, minority groups (racial/ethnic and sexual minorities), and those who have experienced stressful childhood and lifetime events. These patients will become part of your lens as you instinctively offer care in a trauma-informed manner, with ease, competence, and tools to lessen pain.

ORGANIZATION OF THE BOOK

What you'll discover in this discussion is both basic and advanced information about trauma and how we as nurses have much to offer in overcoming trauma's legacy. Nurses are consistently rated as the highest trusted professionals for ethics and honesty (Brenan, 2018), and our hope is that this book will support continuation of this trust. We have organized this book's initial content in Chapter 1 to provide a foundation of what psychological trauma is and its physical, developmental, and emotional manifestations. The reactions of our brains to such fear-inducing situations and events explain much in future behaviors. Next, we move on to how trauma impacts the ability to learn and function, and we further emphasize how an individual successfully navigates herself in society. Behaviors that are born from trauma can be easily misinterpreted. Once those narratives are in place, they are difficult to amend. The heart of this book, however, revolves around specific strategies to increase your awareness of life experiences that include trauma and traumatic events, as an individual and as a nurse.

In Chapter 2, we examine trauma as you become a nurse and the unique aspects of the nursing profession that interface with psychological trauma. We provide information so that you can recognize signs and symptoms of trauma to support your journey in becoming a nurse. Myriad types of trauma, unfortunately, invade nursing today. From historical trauma, passed down from generation to generation, to workplace violence, nurses need to be ready and prepared to face these phenomena.

In Chapters 3 and 4, we discuss ways to assess for psychological injuries and specific strategies to heal from trauma. We discuss how adverse experiences in childhood impact individuals' health and mortality. As well, we provide an overview of the experience, event, and effects of trauma, important considerations for individuals as they interpret the meaning of the trauma in their lives. In these chapters, principles of trauma-informed care and how nurses' different forms of knowledge can address trauma are emphasized. Lastly, we offer advice on how nurses can use information from trauma-informed approaches to provide effective interventions to those who have experienced trauma.

This brings us to Chapter 5, in which education and healthcare organizations can integrate trauma awareness and practices. Existing guidelines are mapped to trauma-informed principles for educators and supervisors. Moving from systems to individual practices in Chapter 6, we present ways the new nurse can promote healing in patients through the use of theory and the ways of knowing in nursing. In Chapter 7, we describe how trauma may be situated in the legal and ethical environments, carved by federal laws and an awareness of violence against women and men, particularly in academic settings. We examine the vulnerabilities of those whose sexual and gender identifications lay outside of mainstream ideologies.

We summarize our discussion in the final chapter, and with your new self-awareness, leave you with thoughts to consider as you move closer to becoming a professional nurse. Through a delineation of the trends reflected in this body of work, we discuss what we see for the future shaped by a trauma-informed view. Our hope is for you to become more resilient and more compassionate and to deliver higher quality care with the knowledge provided in this book.

A word about the evidence we cite in this text. Many individuals believe that literature published longer than five years ago is outdated. While we agree with this rule the majority of the time, we take a slightly different view in this book for a number of reasons. First, the discovery of new knowledge is cumulative. At times, there may not be more recent literature to cite; therefore, an older publication still offers new, relevant information. This may be a seminal paper, influencing later work, or simply knowledge that no other piece of published work can replace. Second, we take an interdisciplinary approach to the literature cited in this book. As trauma is continually and increasingly studied in various disciplines, including nursing, we needed to ensure that the best information was included, regardless of the discipline of origin. Third, while our goal has been to present an overview of trauma, the literature far surpasses what our space in this book allows. Given this, we have attempted to include systematic review articles, meta-synthesis and meta-analysis, and other "state of the science" reviews. In other words, these articles provide rigorous summaries of the published literature on the topic. The student nurse and new nurse are encouraged to pursue additional study as needs and interests direct.

We also interject "Trauma-Informed Reflections." These questions may be the basis for individual, paired, or group reflections and discussions. They coincide with the subject being discussed and provide opportunities for you to expand on the topic. The questions are meant to bring a deeper understanding of the content, more than the consumption of knowledge brings us.

One last thought to share with you. Companion books accompany this text: an instructor's guide and student workbook. These supplementary texts offer activities and simulations that allow application of the content of this "parent" book. As with the narratives presented in this book, each simulation is based on composite cases, representing no one individual, but a conglomeration of vignettes to facilitate application of trauma-informed care. You may recognize yourself, a family member, a peer, or a friend in the accompanying student workbook's simulation case studies. These cases reside in our academic and practice environments, in individuals and patients whose paths cross ours, bound together by trauma.

As we close this introduction, we'd like to leave you with another quote from Gandhi—one that speaks to what we believe to be a critical part of person-centered care. As data science and technology construct important paradigms in healthcare today, we want to remind you that it is the humanness we bring to those under our care and to ourselves that brings us healing. We discuss compassion at length in this book, but for now, it is an important reminder.

> *"Compassion is a muscle that gets stronger with use."*
>
> – Mahatma Gandhi

REFERENCE

Brenan, M. (20 December, 2018). Nurses again outpace other professions for honesty, ethics. *Gallup*. Retrieved from https://news.gallup.com/poll/245597/nurses-again-outpace-professions-honesty-ethics.aspx

LEARNING OBJECTIVES

At the end of this chapter, you will be able to:

- Compare "trauma" to "psychological trauma" and "trauma nursing" to "trauma in nursing."
- Articulate the definition of trauma provided by the Substance Abuse and Mental Health Services Administration (SAMHSA, 2014).
- Break down the brain's anatomical and physiological reactions to chronic stress and traumatic events.
- Categorize how trauma and dose-dependent adverse childhood experiences (ACEs) may affect an individual's morbidity and mortality.
- Describe classifications of trauma, including acute, chronic, complex, and developmental.
- Define various types of trauma specific to professional nurses, including secondary trauma/compassion fatigue/vicarious trauma, second-victim trauma, historical trauma, treatment trauma, and trauma from disasters.
- Discuss the global crisis of childhood abuse and neglect within a framework of trauma.

UNDERSTANDING PSYCHOLOGICAL TRAUMA

1

PURPOSE OF THE CHAPTER

What is psychological trauma? How is it different from being scared or un-comfortable? How is psychological trauma distinct from the trauma we see sensationalized in videos and real-time social media? Indeed, there is even a specialization in nursing called "trauma nursing," which represents many life-threatening patient scenarios that occur in emergency departments (EDs) across the country. We envision immediate rescue efforts; without those efforts, the patient will surely die. In this chapter, we look at life-threatening trauma and compare it to psychological trauma. We discuss different classi-fications of trauma so that at the end of this chapter, your trauma lexicon will be expanded, and you'll be well on your way to being a trauma-informed pro-vider. In Chapter 2, we expand the conversation to examine trauma unique to nurses and the nursing profession.

TRAUMA IN SOCIETY

It seems in today's society, it's not *if* you have experienced trauma or been exposed to another's trauma, but when, under what circumstances, and how frequently. Based upon our education and interactions with those who have traumatic events in their pasts, understanding the individual processes and recovery is the paramount objective. But getting from Point A (trauma) to Point Z (healing) can be like trying to find a path in dry, deep sand, challenging our balance and creating new discomfort. Social norms influence our path: We are suddenly sullied by the actions of others. We wonder about our culpability. Words become important; the language we use, therefore, creates a reality by which to live and ask others to live in.

In the important work by Judith Herman, *Trauma and Recovery* (2015; originally published in 1992), she describes the phenomenon between expression of injury and the secrecy intertwined with such injuries:

> The ordinary response to atrocities is to banish them from consciousness. Certain violations of the social compact are too terrible to utter aloud: this is the meaning of the word unspeakable. (p. 1)

This balance between expression and keeping our secrets hidden often characterizes those of us who have been terribly hurt. We feel we burden others and risk too much if we speak about our secrets, and dozens of reasons arise to prevent us from speaking:

"It was probably my fault, too."

"I should be stronger."

"Why do these things happen to me? It must be me."

While there may be no answer to why it happened, there can be answers to many of our other questions. Within this context, there is intentional and unintentional trauma. As individuals and nurses, we may experience both:

- Bullying, in real time, in real space, and cyber-bullying

- Deaths and accidents of close family, friends, and patients
- Suicide and other disabling mental illnesses
- Psychological and physical neglect and abuse
- Natural disasters
- School shootings
- Personal violence, such as assault and rape
- Ongoing financial stressors and overwhelming debt
- Threats of, and actual, global warfare
- Earth's changing climate and forecasts of future endangerment to the population

This list portrays just some of the potential sources of trauma we experience in today's society. These experiences may be firsthand or come from witnessing the trauma of others.

TRAUMA NURSING

A respected journal, *Journal of Trauma Nursing,* published by Wolters Kluwer, is the official journal of the Society of Trauma Nurses. Nurses may specialize in trauma nursing and, through the Board of Certification for Emergency Nursing, may become a Trauma Certified Registered Nurse (TCRN). Trauma centers in hospitals are frequently cited as locations where the injured are taken after a serious motor vehicle accident and where patients are transferred for emergency care. These centers are designated by levels based on the resources available and the number of patients admitted annually. In this context, trauma encompasses physical, emergent cases where patients have experienced life-threatening injuries. While trauma in this context may encompass psychological trauma, typically the primary focus on trauma nursing is care rendered to save the life of a patient who is in need of emergency care.

This book slices off an important part of this larger trauma concept and zeros in on the psychological trauma that accompanies such physical trauma or exists separately from such a physical experience. Henceforth in the text, when we refer to "trauma," we are referencing psychological trauma, as opposed to sudden, life-threatening (physical) trauma. Figure 1.1 depicts the types of trauma, the way trauma has both a neurobiological component and a human interpretive aspect, and the nurse's interface within this conceptual model. The two circles at the bottom of the figure depict a conceptual distinction between individual and nurse-societal related traumas. It is important to see how these circles overlap, indicating that a person may experience traumas on both sides of our circle. The circle also represents the fluidity and nonlinearity of trauma.

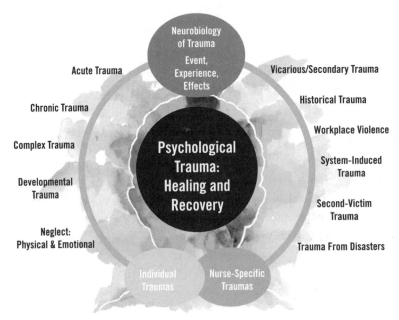

FIGURE 1.1   Conceptualizing trauma.

TRAUMA: THE BASICS

If not referencing a life-threatening physical traumatic injury, what is trauma? In this context, trauma is being exposed to or experiencing a distressing event so that you feel extreme anguish or a sense of being unsafe. This distress may, of course, accompany physical injury. And physical trauma or disability can feed into and be a part of psychological trauma. The subsequent reaction may include myriad psychological outcomes, such as internalizing behaviors (for example, anxiety or depression) or externalizing behaviors (for example, acting out, aggression, emotional dysregulation), and includes posttraumatic stress disorder (PTSD). Nurses' clinical mental model of trauma is often associated with codes or significant physical injury that is life threatening, sudden, and unexpected. A different yet related aspect to such injury, psychological trauma, invades our society. No human being is exempt from traumatic events, and the way trauma is addressed often dictates future successes and challenges. Psychological trauma, symptoms of experiencing traumatic events, and the disorders that sometimes follow thread into aspects of an individual's existence in society.

The Substance Abuse and Mental Health Services Administration (SAMHSA), a government agency within the US Department of Health and Human Services, refers to trauma as:

> experiences that cause intense physical and psychological stress reactions. It can refer to a single event, multiple events, or a set of circumstances that is experienced by an individual as physically and emotionally harmful or threatening and that has lasting adverse effects on the individual's physical, social, emotional, or spiritual well-being. (SAMHSA, 2014, n.p.)

So, let's deconstruct this definition. First, we have an intense reaction to an experience or event. In other words, it is not the type of stress reaction you experience as you sit down to take a routine test in a class or engage in conflict with your best friend. Second, in circumstances involving trauma, the individual has a lasting reaction to that experience. And with that lasting reaction, an individual's life may be affected in adverse ways, experiencing PTSD. This is an example of how an earlier traumatic experience continues to affect the individual's life after the initial exposure to the trauma.

POSTTRAUMATIC STRESS DISORDER AND POSTTRAUMATIC STRESS SYMPTOMS

What happens to an individual after trauma? This is the main question we address in this book, but individual accounts of the aftermath from psychological trauma can be located in ancient literature as retelling of events (Birmes, Hatton, Brunet, & Schmitt, 2003). These accounts evolved into more formal descriptions after the Civil War and early railway accidents in the 19th century. However, World War I triggered the development of medical and psychological theories of how traumatic events affected the lives of those who had experienced such events (Birmes et al., 2003).

Trauma evokes stress; we have a stress response when exposed to trauma. Hans Selye's work on stress and our reactions to it link our mind and body responses. It began with a one-page letter to *Nature* in 1936 in which Selye described stress and how the body adapted to it. At the other end of his four-decade career, at the age of 68, Selye (1976) wrote *Stress in Health and Disease,* an encyclopedia of knowledge and "panoramic overview" (p. 1171) of stress. He wrote:

> At the present period of history, stress in health and disease is medically, sociologically and philosophically the most meaningful subject for humanity that I can think of. (p. 1171)

Selye's groundbreaking work led many scientists to examine the neurologic, endocrinologic, and metabolic effects of stress, and his findings were the first to classify steroid hormones (Szabo, Tache, & Somogyi, 2012). He was inclusive in approaching how stress affects us and wrote: "Stress is the nonspecific response of the body to any demand" (Selye, 1976, p. 15). Further, stress could emanate from positive as well as negative demands placed on us with two types of stress responses (eustress and distress). He emphasized that stresses didn't differ, but the effects of stress did (Selye, 1976). The General Adaptation Syndrome or GAS (later named *stress response)* consists of three stages: the alarm reaction (initial reaction to the stress), resistance (if the organism survives, it rebounds, resists, or adapts), and finally, exhaustion (resources are depleted; Selye, 1976). Working from animal models, it was the ability to adapt to stress—Selye's work was grounded in the natural sciences—that was key to survival.

Scientific advances have created more questions related to physiological changes, internal and external stressors, and the psychological perceptions of stress. This integration of the biological changes, down to the neural circuit level, and the behavioral/psychological factors that impact the initial stress response form ongoing dialogues. But normal stress isn't the same as that experienced during a traumatic event.

The diagnosis of PTSD ties the phenomena of trauma and stress together: the effects of stress created by trauma. The American Psychiatric Association (APA) outlines diagnostic criteria for PTSD for adults, adolescents, and children older than 6 years of age, as well as for children younger than 6 years, in the *Diagnostic and Statistical Manual of Mental Disorders,* Fifth Edition (DSM-5). For those older than 6 years, the criteria are (APA, 2013, pp. 271–272):

1. Exposure to the threat (direct experience, witnessing an event, learning of a close friend/family member's experience, experiencing repeated or extreme exposure to an event)

2. One or more intrusive symptoms related to the trauma (recurrent, involuntary distressing memories, dreams, or dissociative reactions, such as flashbacks, psychological distress, and physical reactions related to the event)

3. Avoidance of stimuli of the event (evading memories, thoughts, and feelings as well as external reminders)

4. Alterations in mood and cognition after the event (loss of memory regarding the event)

5. Experiencing reactions and arousals associated with the trauma

6. Symptoms lasting for more than one month

7. Functioning that has been impacted (social, occupational, and so on)

8. Symptoms that cannot be attributed to substances or a medical condition

Each individual's PTSD experiences will vary, with some appearing more anxious and others experiencing depressive symptoms. The severity of the symptoms will also vary, but PTSD can occur at any age (APA, 2013).

Posttraumatic stress symptoms (PTSS) are components used to diagnose PTSD. For example, one PTSS that may be assessed is cognitive deficits. In his practice, John often hears college-age students report not being able to focus or think clearly, having difficulty keeping up with course material. In fact, as he establishes a therapeutic relationship with them and they choose to share past traumatic experiences with him, he traces their reports of cognitive difficulties to post trauma rather than attention deficits or other disorders. Often, as the trauma is processed, the individual becomes more aware of what is contributing to the lack of focus, clarity, and concentration. This, in turns, supports improvement in the student's cognitive functioning.

Be aware, however, in addition to PTSD, there are several "trauma- and stress-related disorders" (APA, 2013, p. 265). These include reactive attachment disorder (discussed in the following "Attachment" section), disinhibited social engagement disorder, acute stress disorder, and adjustment disorders (APA, 2013).

THE NEUROBIOLOGY OF TRAUMA: KEY CHANGES IN PHYSIOLOGY AND BEHAVIORS

Imagine an individual whose thoughts are tied to the engine of a small motorboat in a large lake. The vessel is powered by an outboard motor that the individual cannot turn off, except when it is out of gas. No matter how the individual tries to turn the motor off, it cannot be stopped except when resources are depleted. The individual/motor is conditioned to run, even when running isn't necessary any longer. Focusing on a goal, a place to dock is impossible because the boat cannot be stopped. This metaphor is similar to a brain exposed to trauma and locked into a neurocognitive cycle. The physical and psychological become intertwined, and the brain doesn't know how to power down and relax. It consumes resources, and it is exhausting to sustain. This is described by Evans and Coccoma (2014) when emphasizing the importance of fear extinction (a return to baseline functioning when a threat is no longer present):

> When the autoregulation of the stress response system is dysfunctional, persons who experienced traumatic events in the past continue to experience heightened neurochemical reactions in the present without the existence of threat. (p. 21)

Fear extinction, an ability to return to our normal state after a threat is removed, is necessary (Evans & Coccoma, 2014). The lack of such extinction may create enduring symptoms of trauma as well as long-term cognitive, emotional, and physical outcomes. When faced with trauma, our brains react. The hippocampus (memory and cognition), amygdala (over activity impacts fear extinction and impedes rational thinking), and prefrontal cortex (rational thought and meaning of experience) create a symphony of reactions when an individual is faced with short-term stress, prolonged stress, and trauma (Evans & Coccoma, 2014). Studies in youth have found excessive glucocorticoid cortisol levels when PTSS is experienced (Carrion & Wong, 2012). This level, in turn, decreases hippocampal volume and prefrontal cortex volume, which may impact memory and executive functioning (Carrion & Wong, 2012). Implications for emotional regulation, learning, and impulse control are evident.

TOXIC STRESS

The ability to regulate our cognitive, emotional, and social expressions begins to form in our early brains. When young brains are exposed to prolonged and excessive stress, the ability to self-regulate may be impaired. Three responses to stress are possible. The first is a positive stress response, where we are able to process stress, despite a mild elevation in heart rate and hormone levels. The second possible response is a stress response that doesn't overwhelm our systems; it is tolerable with concomitant alerted bodily responses. But the stress is time limited, and typically, the young brain has resources to draw upon, such as competent adults in the environment. The third type of stress, toxic stress, is when the stress is intense, prolonged, and severe. Lifelong impairment may result from such toxic stress (Franke, 2014; Harvard University, 2018).

SELF-REGULATION

When a young child experiences toxic stress, self-regulation may be affected and result in trauma-based psychiatric disorders. These disorders represent the inability to accurately identify the "safety-threat potential" of incoming stimuli (Nicholson, Durand, Vance, McGuinness, & Carpenter, 2018). This inaccuracy of interpreting information in our environment may result in the individuals' inability to effectively navigate their world. Their brains may be primed to a survival mode with cardiovascular and cortical/sub-cortical networks being adversely affected. This is in contrast to flexibly and accurately processing people, tasks, and situations surrounding them (Nicholson et al., 2018). Thus, the motorboat's engine is primed to keep running. With our heightened sense of how the brain and body react to toxic stress, refined diagnoses and interventions are possible.

We've discussed toxic stress in the preceding section and its effects on children, with particular attention paid to the influence of such stress in adulthood. The intensity and chronicity of adverse conditions characterize this type of trauma that produces toxicity and allostatic load within an individual. This type of prolonged adverse condition results in an altered stress response characterized by dysregulation and maladaptive coping. Such prevalent stress, originating in childhood but lingering through adulthood, has effects not only on the individual but also on communities and society. A theoretical framework has been forwarded by scholars in public health (Shern, Blanch, & Steverman, 2016) who attribute the current public health crisis to toxic stress:

> The experience of and reaction to toxic stress may provide an organizing framework for understanding how these social influences operate and for mounting a comprehensive public health response. (p. 112)

Positioning toxic stress as a framework for public health might offer us better strategies to combat several health crises facing society today. These include chronic diseases (for example, cancer, cardiovascular disease, and diabetes) as well as broader, more informed approaches to what are considered by many to be behavioral choices (for example, substance use, obesity, and sexually transmitted diseases).

ATTACHMENT

As we discuss trauma broadly, a more detailed description of how trauma may affect attachment is necessary. For adults, it may be distrusting others, continuing to hide secrets, being unable to form stable and healthy relationships, and turning inward from the world. In the world of adoption and foster care, approaches to secure attachments with caregivers are abundant, particularly so when trauma is in the child's or adolescent's past. The DSM-5 (APA, 2013) discusses two disorders in particular related to children: reactive attachment disorder and disinhibited social engagement disorder:

- Reactive attachment disorder is considered relatively rare. It may be caused from severe neglect or children being placed in institutions, such as those found in Eastern Europe in the past decades. In these instances, the child rarely seeks or is able to receive comfort when distressed.

- Disinhibited social engagement disorder is also thought to be rare. It may occur due to severe neglect or from being raised in institutional settings, such as orphanages. In essence, the child doesn't seem to discriminate within cultural and social norms of approaching and interacting with adults. The child may demonstrate overly familiar verbal or physical behavior with strangers.

For both disorders, the lack of typical attachment behaviors (inhibited or exaggerated and indiscriminate) is evident.

TRAUMA AND THE EFFECTS ON THE BODY

As nurses, we believe in approaching the individual as a whole being, a multidimensional person with psychological, physical, emotional, social, and spiritual facets. As part of this belief, we understand that the person acts as a system, with one dimension influencing the others. Extending this concept and within this context, evidence supports that the experience of trauma has major implications on health and longevity. In Chapter 3, we discuss adverse childhood experiences, which carry the significant risk of trauma, and the adverse health implications of these events early in life. Here, we'd like to emphasize how potentially damaging trauma can be—even influencing mortality. (See Figure 1.2.)

Researchers have looked at this relationship at the level of our DNA. Human telomeres, DNA protein structures, are biomarkers used as proxies to examine life expectancies and age-related diseases. Several theories have been proposed as to why telomere length is shortened in the presence of trauma, including the production of destructive radicals and molecules, chronic inflammation, and co-occurring psychiatric disorders. In an overview, Price, Kao, Burgers, Carpenter, and Tyrka (2013) explain how telomere length is associated with various diseases and experiences. They use insightful questions surrounding the hypothesized relationships between early life stress and shortened telomere lengths. Their overview emphasizes how this area of research has surged as research questions are refined (Price et al., 2013). Thus, to determine whether telomere length is associated with PTSD, Li, Wang, Zhou, Huang, and Li (2017) conducted a meta-analysis that compiled data from 3,851 patients in five studies. Across gender groups, PTSD was associated with shorter telomere lengths. Specific groups were also analyzed: Diminished telomere lengths were found for those individuals who had experienced sexual assault and childhood trauma (Li et al., 2017).

Evidence now suggests that our genes may be affected by childhood adversity. Papale, Seltzer, Madrid, Pollak, and Alisch (2018) collected salivary samples from 22 girls, ranging in age between 9 and 12 years, and compared gene expressions between those who had experienced normative and high stress exposure. Not only did the researchers find that the girls who had experienced high stress demonstrated more behavioral problems, but they discovered 122 differentially methylated genes were associated with the high stress group (Papale et al., 2018). Obviously, more scientific studies are needed; however, these findings present us with evidence of the link between negative social exposure and neuromolecular changes at the genetic level.

TRAUMA AND LEARNING

Traumatic stress has implications in multiple areas of functioning. We now understand how the body reacts to stress and how these reactions affect our brain. When a brain is engaged in decoding danger, how can it be open to learning? Neurodevelopmental scientists have identified two areas that are affected when traumatic stress and posttraumatic stress are experienced: areas related to executive functioning and memory (Carrion & Wong, 2012). Think about patient education, discharge planning, and care coordination. If an individual is in a state of posttraumatic stress, how much will that individual absorb and retain?

ADDITIONAL TRAUMA EFFECTS ON OUR PHYSICAL HEALTH

Reports of physical health complaints are not uncommon among trauma survivors. One aspect that affects our health is the quality and quantity of sleep we get. The regenerative properties of sleep are well known. However, sleep hygiene for trauma survivors may be challenging. Miller, Jaffe, Davis, Pruiksma, and Rhudy (2015) studied the relationships between sleep disturbances, PTSD, depression, and physical health. Reported findings in a regression analysis included that sleep disturbances were related to physical health problems over what would be expected by PTSD and depressive symptoms alone; therefore, sleep disturbances appear to be a predictor of physical health problems in those who have experienced trauma (Miller et al., 2015). Although the study had a modest sample ($n =$ 54), sleep quality should be assessed by caregivers.

A groundbreaking study conducted by Felitti et al. (1998) uncovered the connection between ACEs and adult morbidity and mortality. We discuss this study in more detail in Chapter 3, but this research drew attention to the dose-dependent way (the higher the individual's ACE score, the greater the effect on the body) childhood experiences, such as abuse and neglect, affect our health. Figure 1.2 presents how adults with greater than 6 (out of 10) ACEs had on average 20 years less life expectancy and staggering economic costs to society (Felitti et al., 1998).

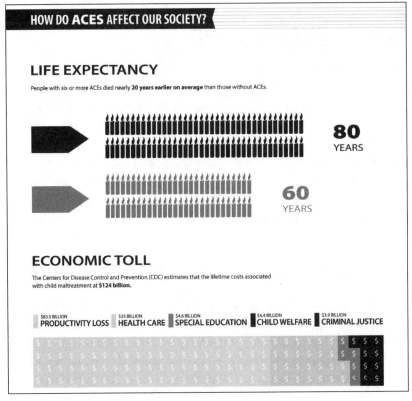

FIGURE 1.2   How do ACEs affect our society?

Source: Centers for Disease Control and Prevention, n.d.

As Figure 1.2 shows, the load of six or more ACEs denied those individuals two decades of life that were available, on average, to those with fewer ACE scores. Lost productivity, increased healthcare costs, special education resources, child welfare, and costs of the criminal justice system have all been traced to childhood maltreatment for a total of $124 billion. In the "Trauma in the Shadows" sidebar, we share a narrative of a nursing student reminded of past childhood maltreatment and how it became an unwelcome part of her current life.

TRAUMA IN THE SHADOWS

Fall was her favorite time of year, and the beginning of the first semester of her junior year made Gabriella feel that she was close to achieving her life goal of becoming a nurse. Gabriella's excitement to enter into her public health course was, in part, due to her mother's love of making a difference in her community. She considered her mother something of a hero, a woman who had returned to college after escaping an abusive relationship with Gabriella's father, long absent from the family. Her mom had gone on to become the director of a nonprofit center for non-English speaking residents in the community. They would laugh about how they didn't need anyone outside the family—her mom and her two daughters—to get through life. Gabriella wanted to be just like her.

Today was Gabriella's first clinical day, and she and her friend, Chelsey, were driving to the clinic that administered the Special Supplemental Nutrition Program for Women, Infants, and Children. She was to shadow and assist the nurse who counseled breastfeeding mothers on proper nutrition. They arrived and left their backpacks in the car, taking only a pen and some materials for the assignment based on their field experiences.

Gabriella's morning went smoothly. She enjoyed helping the nurse as she discussed the significant advantages of breastfeeding and food choices that would benefit both the mom and the baby. After the third mom had left, Gabriella went to call the next mom in line. She froze. The mother carried a small infant, with only a diaper on, and a toddler in tow. The woman must have been in her mid-twenties, and had a blackened eye and swollen lip. Her hair color was the same color as Gabriella's mother when she was a young mother. The toddler, a small girl, had the same eyes as Gabriella's older sister.

Gabriella returned to the nurse alone. The nurse looked at her confused and asked, "Where is the next mom?"

Gabriella felt as if she was suddenly in a dream, unable to focus on her surroundings. An image appeared in her mind, but it, too, was fuzzy and seemed to jump in and out of her consciousness. She felt as if she couldn't breathe enough to oxygenate her body, resulting in lightheadedness. She found a chair and sat down. Finally, she mumbled something and said, "I don't feel well. Can I leave?"

The nurse nodded and said, "Are you OK to drive? You look really pale. Did you eat breakfast?"

"I'm fine. Just a little queasy. Let me tell my friend I'm leaving." Gabriella told Chelsey that she needed to leave as soon as possible. Her friend looked at her and immediately reassured her that she could arrange for a ride home.

Back in her dorm room and for the rest of the day, Gabriella chided herself and worried about her clinical instructor's reaction to her leaving the clinic so suddenly. When she was able to contact her instructor, she tried to describe how she felt, but she was having difficulty. The instructor was understanding but encouraged Gabriella to get "checked out" if the symptoms continued. She advised her to keep a food diary to see whether her symptoms were related to food intake and blood sugar levels.

When she arrived at the dining court for dinner, the noise overwhelmed her. She scanned the room that was full of college students eating. She kept looking around with a heightened sense of some unknown urgency as she surveyed each group of people. She tried to convince herself that it was just like every night had been for the past two years that she'd lived there. But she couldn't shake the feeling of panic and not feeling safe. After a short time, she left and went back to her room.

That night, Gabriella's dreams were of her home and shadows. Screams and shouts, but not from her. She called her mom after a night of panic and confusion. She described what had happened at the clinic and last night. After a long sigh, her mother whispered, "I'm so sorry, honey." She went on to describe how Gabriella was only a little over 3 years old when the violence had escalated. Yes, her mother had had a black eye and a bloodied mouth, both prompting her to obtain a restraining order and live in a shelter for a few days, until she moved in with a friend with her two young daughters. She apologized for the chaos that had surrounded Gabriella at such a young age. They continued to talk for another hour, Gabriella missing another class.

The next two weeks were a blur, with Gabriella sinking further into a "funk." But she was also nervous, unable to relax, and vigilant in crowds. She began to avoid her chemistry class, taught by an older man. She'd cut off contact with many friends and even began to avoid her mother's calls. Gabriella began to overeat and ordered food delivery, charging hundreds of dollars. She just wanted to feel safe and in control again but didn't think it was a big deal. Her grades started to drop, and by mid-semester, she was failing two courses.

When Gabriella opened her mail and saw the formal letter from the university cautioning her that she may be on academic probation if she didn't raise her grades, she realized something had happened to her and she needed to find out what that was. One of her friends had described a group he belonged to for students diagnosed with attention deficit issues. The services were offered through the university-based counseling center. She decided to call for an appointment.

Gabriella was informed that she would be triaged and assessed for services in a face-to-face meeting. After the intake coordinator assessed her symptoms, she was referred to have a more formal intake for individual counseling. The therapist, Hannah, was a middle-aged female and a trauma-informed provider. She promised Gabriella that the environment was safe and that their interactions were sacred to her.

The sessions were intense, and Gabriella worked hard to gain insight into what had happened to her—how that day in the clinic had triggered past traumatic events and how it had affected her today as a young adult. She grieved and allowed herself to feel the emotions that had been experienced before she could verbalize them. The sessions exhausted her, and the work was difficult. She managed to pass her fall courses and register for another semester. With several months of therapy behind her, Gabriella began to feel centered, more competent, and less anxious. She was again looking forward to achieving her life goal of becoming a nurse.

Gabriella's story reflects early trauma, when the child may be unable to verbalize the sense of terror and foreboding surrounding maltreatment. Her young adult behaviors were goal oriented, even if initially maladaptive. They make sense when the context of trauma is considered with the need to feel safe and in control of the environment.

TRAUMA AND PTSD: VULNERABLE GROUPS

Some individuals are vulnerable to developing PTSD after being exposed to traumatic events. While certain groups are identified in this section, it is the *exposure* that makes them susceptible to PTSD and increases their risk of negative outcomes, including suicide. For example, those individuals who are exposed to natural or man-made disasters may be more susceptible to PTSD. As a nurse, you need to be mindful of demographic, social, and occupational risk factors that place individuals in harm's way more often than others. Groups who are particularly vulnerable to PTSD include veterans, police, firefighters, and first responders, such as emergency medical personnel (APA, 2013). At the highest risk of experiencing PTSD are those individuals who have survived interpersonal violence, such as "rape, military combat and captivity, and ethnically or politically motivated internment or genocide" (APA, 2013, p. 276).

Females experience more PTSD, and with longer durations. This evidence is predicated on the fact that females often experience more traumatic events (for example, rape and assault) than males. However, when groups with similar exposures are compared, gender as a risk factor becomes nonsignificant (APA, 2013). Preliminary evidence supports that childhood abuse predicts female-perpetrated psychological and physical dating violence (Kendra, Bell, & Guimond, 2012). The researchers also found a positive relationship between child abuse, dating violence, and anger arousal. Speculation about misinterpreting partners' reactions (overly hostile) may trigger an anger arousal and thus, correlate with dating violence (Kendra et al., 2012).

Ethnicity and race also seem to affect some groups more than others, with higher reports of PTSD in US Latinos, African Americans, and American Indians/Native Americans (APA, 2013). Environmental and social factors such as social determinants may impact prevalence rates of PTSD. Sexual minority individuals and individuals with cognitive and/or physical disabilities may be vulnerable to psychological and physical trauma. Children in households with impaired caregivers or caregivers with mental health impairment (or both) are also at higher risk for frequent trauma as well as neglect (Vivrette et al., 2018). Emphasis on the individual nature of the stress reactions to trauma is important; such individual responses are influenced by genetic predispositions, support systems, and the type, intensity, and duration of the trauma.

While our mental models of psychological injury link us to these vulnerable groups, we need to state with certainty that trauma affects all members in society: those with affluence and those without; those in ethnic and racial majorities and minorities. Trauma cuts across genders, and assumptions and stereotypes based on social strata are misguided. Our belief holds that:

> It is a myth that those born into privilege do not experience trauma; it is also a fallacy that those who have been neglected, abused or bereaved will automatically become deeply damaged adults. (Rahim, 2014, p. 554)

Nurses are in pivotal positions to enter into patient interactions without biases or assumptions. Trauma is experienced and processed at an individual level, influenced by myriad factors. Assumptions obfuscate quality care.

TYPES OF TRAUMA

Experts have classified the various types of trauma and how each can influence an individual. Table 1.1 outlines the types of trauma and categorizes them into individual-focused or nurse-other-focused traumas (discussed in Chapter 2). Note that these categories are fluid and serve to provide structure to the discussion. Assorted arguments could be made for a different categorization on several trauma types.

TABLE 1.1 TYPES OF TRAUMA AND ACTORS INVOLVED

TYPES OF TRAUMA	INDIVIDUAL-FOCUSED	NURSE-OTHER-FOCUSED
Acute trauma	✺	
Chronic trauma	✺	
Complex trauma/Interpersonal trauma	✺	
Developmental trauma	✺	
Neglect (physical and psychological)	✺	
Vicarious trauma/Secondary trauma*		✹
Second-victim trauma*		✹
Workplace violence*		✹
Historical trauma*		✹
Treatment trauma/System-induced trauma*		✹
Trauma from disasters*		✹

Discussed in Chapter 2

ACUTE TRAUMA

Acute trauma is similar to an acute physical event. It occurs as a single event for a limited time. Examples may include rape, physical assault (for nurses, this includes workplace violence, which we talk about in Chapter 2), a contained natural disaster, and accidents involving modes of transportation (cars, trains, airplanes, and so on). As you can surmise, acute trauma may vary in terms of the amount of intimate trauma experienced and whether the trauma was intentionally inflicted.

CHRONIC TRAUMA

Chronic trauma is sustained, repeated, and prolonged. For example, chronic trauma may be experienced by a mother and her children who live with an abusive spouse/parent or significant other for years or children who experience bullying from peers over the course of high school. The length of the chronic trauma varies, but its duration may be years. The day-in-day-out knowing that exposure will come to the individual creates fear, shame, and helplessness. Children in the foster care system who have been removed from their birthparents' home due to abuse and/or neglect and have had multiple placements with different foster caregivers have often experienced chronic trauma.

COMPLEX TRAUMA/INTERPERSONAL TRAUMA

Closely connected with developmental trauma (see the next section) are those children who have experienced trauma, usually by those trusted caregivers and family members, to provide for their physical and emotional needs. Often, the effects of complex/interpersonal trauma are especially adversely impactful to the individual. Caregivers whom the child trusts, who should be fulfilling a promise of nurturing and protection, have betrayed the child's trust and society's moral and legal laws and have themselves become the perpetrators of psychological injury.

DEVELOPMENTAL TRAUMA

Although excluded as a diagnostic category in the DSM-5 (APA, 2013), a developmental trauma framework captures the phenomenon of prolonged trauma during childhood development that negatively impacts typical psychological growth. Children and youth who do not experience developmental trauma are raised by caregivers—usually parents—who provide consistency, competency, and nurturing. Developmental milestones are met, barring other conditions, and the individual progresses toward adulthood with the ability to establish connections with others and feel competent in life. For those who have experienced developmental trauma, forming attachments with others may be difficult. Rahim (2014) advocates for a wider discussion of developmental trauma so that interventions can be focused on actual trauma versus symptoms of trauma, such as anxiety, and for recognizing the skewed relationships in adulthood that can result from trauma. In a study of more than 16,000 children and adolescents in the Illinois welfare system who had experienced interpersonal trauma, Kisiel and colleagues (2014) found that the complexity of the trauma resulted in a high level of impairment. The team separated violent and nonviolent interpersonal trauma and found that those who had experienced both were more likely to suffer from increasing difficulties and PTSS (Kisiel et al., 2014). Examining such complex, chronic interpersonal trauma from a developmental framework can result in a clearer understanding of the impact of such trauma and of interventions to address the needs of those affected.

POLY-VICTIMIZATION

Unfortunately, children and adolescents often experience multiple types of traumatic events. In a nationally representative study of 4,053 children and adolescents, poly-victimization (such as sexual assault, child physical abuse, and bullying) was more highly related to trauma symptoms than repeated, single-type victimization (Turner, Finkelhor, & Ormrod, 2010). Turner and colleagues (2010) also found that 66% of the children experienced more than one type of victimization. These findings create avenues for future research, including whether poly-victimizations occur, at times, because of susceptibility created by the initial trauma.

CHILD MALTREATMENT: A FOUNTAIN OF TRAUMA

The American Academy of Pediatrics (AAP) has published several reports and papers on the effects of childhood adversity. One technical report stands out in describing the lasting effects of early adverse childhood events and toxic stress. In this report, Shonkoff and colleagues (2012) argue that the mechanisms of childhood toxic stress create lifelong disruptions, which result in health disparities in adulthood. Further, the AAP views adult disorders that originated from toxic stress as developmental disorders (Shonkoff et al., 2012). Nature—including epigenetics—interacting with nurture throughout the life span allows us to situate the environment in a new way. Adults who themselves experienced toxic stress may be less able to competently parent their children; thus, they are at risk for perpetuating a cycle of intergenerational trauma (see Chapter 2). Efforts at the primary care level may hold promise for shifting the focus from treatment to prevention.

ABUSE: A GLOBAL CRISIS

The World Health Organization (WHO, 2018) estimates that, based on international studies, 25% of all adults report having been physically abused as children. Further, 1 in 5 women and 1 in 13 men report having been sexually abused as a child. In the United States, the incidence and prevalence of child maltreatment (all types of abuse and neglect) are as concerning; see the "Four Common Types of Abuse" sidebar. In 2014 (Child Trends, 2016):

- 702,000 cases of child maltreatment were reported.

- Children 3 years and younger had the higher incidence of maltreatment when compared with older children.

- Reports of neglect were higher than other forms of maltreatment.

- Black, American Indian, Alaskan Native, and multiple-race children had the highest rate of childhood maltreatment.

FOUR COMMON TYPES OF ABUSE

- Physical abuse is the use of intentional physical force, such as hitting, kicking, shaking, burning, or other shows of force against a child.
- Sexual abuse involves engaging a child in sexual acts. It includes fondling, rape, and exposing a child to other sexual activities.
- Emotional abuse refers to behaviors that harm a child's self-worth or emotional well-being. Examples include name calling, shaming, rejecting, withholding love, and threatening.
- Neglect is the failure to meet a child's basic needs. These needs include housing, food, clothing, education, and access to medical care.

Source: Centers for Disease Control and Prevention, 2014

NEGLECT

Neglect is often associated with the absence of care during childhood; however, there is also spousal neglect and the neglect found in older adult abuse. Child neglect may be difficult to define and categorize, yet it is the most common form of maltreatment of children, with 74.8% of investigated cases including neglect (US Department of Health & Human Services, 2018). The impact of neglect is real, yet the evidence occupies a negative space in that it's the absence of care and nurturing. For example:

- It's not having clean clothes.

- It's not receiving praise and acceptance.

- It's not having enough food to eat or a safe place to live.

- It's not having your parent(s) available and not having care provided in their absence.

But neglect can be subtle as well, leaving the individual feeling as if no one cares enough to provide for her emotional and psychological needs; therefore, she must be unworthy of such care and love. Childhood neglect may leave a person believing there is something wrong with her. The APA states that child neglect "results in, or has reasonable potential to result, in psychological harm to the child" (2013, p. 718).

As the individual grows into young adulthood and beyond, such psychological harm may not be at a conscious level. Her self-esteem is damaged, but in a way that escapes her. After all, how is an individual supposed to know what she didn't receive? The typical care offered to children cannot be known to the individual except through other actors in her life, such as extended family, friends, and peers. Her primary source of nurturing cannot offer her a model of care. But this skewed model is what is available to her, and with this model is a transferred belief in its replication.

In the seminal work of Alice Miller (2007), the experiences of the child who has been abused and neglected are deconstructed and analyzed. While Miller (2007) excludes those who have endured extreme abuse and neglect, her primary thesis is that adults who have experienced "desertion" (p. 5) may grow up to believe their childhood was "happy and protected" (p. 5). This illusion is unsustainable, as many experience depression, anxiety, and other internalized and externalized behaviors in an attempt to fill an emotional void. They may continue with this belief and attempt to validate themselves through proving to the world how talented and accomplished they are. This is proof, in their mind, that they are worthy of love: "See! Look at how much I have done! Look at how talented and gifted I am."

Unfortunately, the façade eventually breaks down, and the individual again seeks to find answers based on self-worth. What they value in life and what they believe adds to their value as a person in society. By examining an internal self-worth, divorced from external praise and recognition, the individual will be allowed to claim a right to exist and be of value simply based on humanness.

CONCLUSIONS

This chapter provides a foundation to understanding trauma and the resulting toxic stress that can affect individuals across the life span. Different types of trauma allow us to see the contexts, both physical and temporal, that psychological injury can take. The balance of nature and nurture helps us realize as people and caregivers that trauma is interpreted, experienced, and processed at the individual level. The global crisis of childhood maltreatment creates an urgency for us to understand traumatic events. Neglect—common and complex and a form of maltreatment—drives individuals to seek self-worth through external and internal sources.

HIGHLIGHTS OF CHAPTER CONTENT

- Psychological trauma is defined by SAMHSA (2014) to include experiences that cause intense reactions and create lasting effects.

- Posttraumatic stress disorder (PTSD) and posttraumatic stress symptoms (PTSS) help us diagnose those who suffer the effects of past psychological or physical injuries (APA, 2013).

- Changes in the brain when exposed to stress and trauma may negatively influence learning, cognition, emotional regulation, attachment, and other symptoms that may be incorrectly interpreted.

- Fear extinction is needed to return to a normal state after trauma exposure.

- Myriad and negative health symptoms and outcomes may result from toxic stress and traumatic events.

- Certain groups are more vulnerable to traumatic events; however, no individual is immune to experiencing trauma.

- The global crisis of child maltreatment motivates us to provide competent care across the life span to those who have survived trauma.

- The student and new nurse should be familiar with the different causes and types of trauma.

REFERENCES

American Psychiatric Association. (2013). *Diagnostic and statistical manual of mental disorders* (5th ed.). Arlington, VA: Author.

Birmes, P., Hatton, L., Brunet, A., & Schmitt, L. (2003). Early historical literature for posttraumatic symptomatology. *Stress and Health, 19,* 17–26. doi:10.1002/smi.952

Carrion, V. G., & Wong, S. S. (2012). Can traumatic stress alter the brain? Understanding the implications of early trauma on brain development and learning. *Journal of Adolescent Health, 51,* S23–S28. doi:http://dx.doi.org/10.1016/j.jadohealth.2012.04.010

Centers for Disease Control and Prevention. (n.d.). Adverse childhood experiences: Looking at how ACEs affect our lives and society. Retrieved from https://vetoviolence.cdc.gov/apps/phl/resource_center_infographic.html

Centers for Disease Control and Prevention. (2014). Understanding child maltreatment: Fact sheet. National Center for Injury Prevention and Control. Retrieved from https://www.cdc.gov/violenceprevention/pdf/understanding-cm-factsheet.pdf

Child Trends. (2016). Child maltreatment. Retrieved from https://www.childtrends.org/indicators/child-maltreatment

Evans, A., & Coccoma, P. (2014). *Trauma-informed care: How neuroscience influences practice.* East Sussex, UK: Routledge.

Felitti, V. J., Anda, R. F., Nordenberg, D., Williamson, D. F., Spitz, A. M., Edwards, V., . . . Marks, J. S. (1998). Relationship of childhood abuse and household dysfunction to many of the leading causes of death in adults: The Adverse Childhood Experiences (ACE) study. *American Journal of Preventive Medicine, 14*(4), 245–258.

Franke, H. A. (2014). Toxic stress: Effects, prevention and treatment. *Children, 1,* 390–402. doi:10.3390/children1030390

Harvard University. (2018). Toxic stress. Center on the Developing Child. Retrieved from https://developingchild.harvard.edu/science/key-concepts/toxic-stress/

Herman, J. (2015). *Trauma and recovery: The aftermath of violence—From domestic abuse to political terror.* New York, NY: Basic Books.

Kendra, R., Bell, K. M., & Guimond, J. M. (2012). The impact of child abuse history, PTSD symptoms, and anger arousal on dating violence perpetration among college women. *Journal of Family Violence, 27,* 165–175. doi:10.1007/s10896-012-9415-7

Kisiel, C. L., Fehrenbach, T., Torgersen, E., Stolbach, B., McClelland, G., Griffin, G., & Burkman, K. (2014). Constellations of interpersonal trauma and symptoms in child welfare: Implications for a developmental trauma framework. *Journal of Family Violence, 29,* 1–14. doi:10.1007/s10896-013-9559-0

Li, X., Wang, J., Zhou, J., Huang, P., & Li, J. (2017). The association between posttraumatic stress disorder and shorter telomere length: A systematic review and meta-analysis. *Journal of Affective Disorders, 218,* 322–326. doi:http://dx.doi.org/10.1016/j.jad.2017.03.048

Miller, A. (2007). *The drama of the gifted child: The search for the true self.* New York, NY: Basic Books.

Miller, K. E., Jaffe, A. E., Davis, J. L., Pruiksma, K. E., & Rhudy, J. L. (2015). Relationship between self-reported physical health problems and sleep disturbances among trauma survivors: A brief report. *Sleep Health, 1,* 166–168. doi:http://dx.doi.org/10.1016/j.sleh.2015.05.002

Nicholson, W., Durand, S., Vance, D., McGuinness, T., & Carpenter, J. (2018). *Trauma-based disorders and the cardio-neural mechanisms involved in dysfunctional self-regulation.* Paper presented at the 2018 American Psychiatric Nurses Association Preconference.

Papale, L. A., Seltzer, L. J., Madrid, A., Pollak, S. D., & Alisch, R. S. (2018). Differentially methylated genes in saliva are linked to childhood stress. *Scientific Reports, 8*, 10785. doi:10.1038/s41598-018-29107-0

Price, L. H., Kao, H. T., Burgers, D. E., Carpenter, L. L., & Tyrka, A. R. (2013). Telomeres and early-life stress: An overview. *Biological Psychiatry, 73*, 15–23. doi:https://doi.org/10.1016/j.biopsych.2012.06.025

Rahim, M. (2014). Developmental trauma disorder: An attachment-based perspective. *Clinical Child Psychology and Psychiatry, 19*(4), 548–560. doi:10.1177/1359104514534947

Selye, H. (1936). A syndrome produced by diverse nocuous agents. *Nature, 138*(3479), 32.

Selye, H. (1976). History and general outline of the stress concept. Chapter 1 in *Stress in health and disease.* Boston, MA: Butterworths.

Shern, D. L., Blanch, A. K., & Steverman, S. M. (2016). Toxic stress, behavioral health, and the next major era in public health. *American Journal of Orthopsychiatry, 86*(2), 109–123. doi:http://dx.doi.org/10.1037/ort0000120

Shonkoff, J. P., Garner, A. S., & the Committee on Psychosocial Aspects of Child and Family Health, Committee on Early Childhood, Adoption, and Dependent Care, and Section on Developmental and Behavioral Pediatrics. (2012). The lifelong effects of early childhood adversity and toxic stress. *Pediatrics, 129*(1), e232–e246. doi:10.1542/peds.2011-2663

Substance Abuse and Mental Health Services Administration. (Spring 2014). Key terms: Definitions. *SAMHSA News, 22*(2). Retrieved from https://www.samhsa.gov/samhsaNewsLetter/Volume_22_Number_2/trauma_tip/key_terms.html

Szabo, S., Tache, Y., & Somogyi, A. (2012). The legacy of Hans Selye and the origins of stress research: A retrospective 75 years after his landmark brief "letter" to the editor of *Nature. Stress, 15*(5), 472–478. doi:10.3109/10253890.2012.710919

Turner, H. A., Finkelhor, D., & Ormrod, R. (2010). Poly-victimization in a national sample of children and youth. *American Journal of Preventative Medicine, 38*(3), 323–330. doi:10.1016/j.amepre.2009.11.012

US Department of Health & Human Services, Administration for Children and Families, Administration on Children, Youth and Families, Children's Bureau. (2018). *Child maltreatment 2016.* Retrieved from https://www.acf.hhs.gov/sites/default/files/cb/cm2016.pdf

Vivrette, R. L., Briggs, E. C., Lee, R. C., Kenney, K. T., Houston-Armstrong, T. R., Pynoos, R. S., & Kiser, L. J. (2018). Impaired caregiving, trauma exposure, and psychological functioning in a national sample of children and adolescents. *Journal of Child & Adolescent Trauma, 11*(2), 187–196. doi:https://doi.org/10.1007/s40653-016-0105-0

World Health Organization. (2018). Child maltreatment. Retrieved from http://www.who.int/news-room/fact-sheets/detail/child-maltreatment

LEARNING OBJECTIVES

At the end of this chapter, you will be able to:

- Articulate the types of trauma that often are unique to nurses and experienced in the workplace.
- Examine the phenomenon of compassion fatigue and its effects on personal and professional functioning.
- Consider nursing clinical settings and exposure to trauma.
- Offer a rationale for why certain groups in society, including nurses, may experience historical trauma.
- List ways to modify patient environments to minimize treatment trauma.
- Analyze the distinct traumas in the workplace for nurses, from patient assault and second-victim trauma to incivility (horizontal violence).
- Deconstruct the ethical, legal, and safety factors related to secondary trauma in disaster management activities performed by nurses.

TRAUMA AND BECOMING A NURSE 2

PURPOSE OF THE CHAPTER

Now that we've described the various types of trauma that can affect individuals and have a grasp of what each of these means, we turn our attention to trauma that is unique to nurses and other healthcare workers. In this chapter, we discuss types of traumatic experiences within the healthcare context and as we render care to patients. Although nurses are one of the highest-regarded professions, our business is a risky one, leaving us vulnerable to trauma in myriad ways. From the long-term erosion of our spirits due to vicarious experiences with patients' traumatic events to being treated by peers in mean-spirited/hostile ways, nurses are surrounded by trauma.

TRAUMA UNIQUE TO NURSES AND CAREGIVERS

We want to start this chapter with a story about a nurse. This nurse was a role model for new nurses on the inpatient psychiatric unit. Although fairly young with two small children, she was articulate, solid as a leader, and had a calming influence over the other staff members. Yet, when it came time to pass medications, she needed a supervisor to watch her administer certain drugs. Later, she confided to Karen that her license was on probationary status for opioid diversion, in part due to "alarm fatigue" (Sendelbach & Funk, 2013). Her story is one of secondary trauma. After working for years on a pediatric intensive care unit, she began to experience insomnia, anorexia, and hyperarousal due to a trauma trigger. Whenever an alarm or beeping noise would sound, she would be triggered into reliving a past trauma. "You see," she said, "the sound reminds me of a ventilator alarm, of something gone wrong and a young life in my care." When she was discovered for drug diversion (taking medication that was meant for patients), she knew it was time to reclaim her life. Months of therapy ensued, and she agreed to a recovery monitoring agreement with the state board of nursing to save her nursing license. Karen will always remember this nurse, one she looked to for guidance as a new nurse. She was someone whom Karen never would have guessed would be diverting substances. Yet the secondary trauma was too overwhelming for her, and her coping mechanisms were insufficient at the time. Fortunately, her story ends with peace after the crisis and reclaiming her career and personal life. Let's discuss forms of trauma that are specific and relevant to nurses and other healthcare providers.

TRAUMA EXPERIENCED BY NURSES AS CAREGIVERS

Because of the seemingly unending barrage of needs presented by patients, nurses are particularly susceptible to a unique form of psychological fatigue that impacts the ability to provide emotional availability to their patients. This is called *compassion fatigue*. A similar but distinct form of trauma is secondary trauma or vicarious trauma—what the nurse who diverted substances experienced. The nurse, through witnessing or living through others' trauma, may begin to experience secondary posttraumatic stress symptoms (PTSS). In these instances, nurses are not experiencing firsthand trauma but experiencing the symptoms related to having gone through such stress. We believe nurses, and the nursing care that is rendered, create a unique context and even a vulnerability to experiencing compassion fatigue and secondary trauma.

COMPASSION FATIGUE AND SECONDARY TRAUMA

As a nurse, you hear individuals speak in times of crisis about physical and emotional periods of vulnerability, which, over time, with repeated intensity, can leave a caregiver emotionally spent and unable to give to others. We discuss ways to assess for and combat compassion fatigue in Chapters 3 and 4, where we describe paths to restoration and healing. For now, it is important to understand the characteristics of compassion fatigue and the recurrent themes that appear through a description of the literature. A concept analysis serves to help us understand what the term means and what its attributes or characteristics are. In a concept analysis, Coetzee and Klopper (2010) defined compassion fatigue in nursing as:

> a state where the compassionate energy that is expended by nurses has surpassed their restorative processes, with recovery power being lost. All these states manifest with marked physical, social, emotional, spiritual, and intellectual changes that increase in intensity with each progressive state. (p. 237)

The authors describe compassion fatigue as a cumulative process that may eventually exceed the nurse's endurance and restorative abilities (Coetzee & Klopper, 2010). There is a multidimensional quality; compassion fatigue affects many areas of an individual's functioning. We believe compassion fatigue is a possible outcome of secondary trauma, also referred to as vicarious trauma. Secondary traumas are "stress reactions and symptoms resulting from exposure to another individual's traumatic experiences, rather than from exposure to a traumatic event" (Substance Abuse and Mental Health Services Administration [SAMHSA], 2014, para. 2). Secondary trauma isn't unique to nursing; rather, this exposure can be experienced by many in the health professions, as well as first responders and clergy (SAMHSA, 2014).

Compassion, according to Georges (2011), is a complex phenomenon that occurs within a biopower context. It is the "power over life" in healthcare (p. 131). Nondiscursive forms (values we may believe but not vocalize or express), carrying powerful influences, create the unspeakable in nursing: "the creation/maintenance of biopolitical spaces in which compassion—for oneself or one's patients—is rendered severely diminished or impossible" (p. 131). Frequent, unrelenting elements such as social and market forces, conscious withholding of emotion toward patients and students, valuing evidence and empiricism over theoretical understanding, and other factors in today's nursing care and academic environments result in an inability or unwillingness to show compassion to ourselves and others (Georges, 2011). The unspeakable is often assumed, ingrained into our way of thinking so that we forget to question the very foundations of our thoughts and beliefs.

In your career, you will see, smell, and touch reactions to those who have experienced trauma. The hand you are holding may squeeze yours so tightly you are not sure how much longer you can bear it. An utterance from a patient may catch you off guard, so unexpected that you are not sure you heard correctly. You may be in the ED or on a medical/surgical unit or in a long-term care facility. The patient may be in a life-threatening state from an automobile accident, or hemorrhaging post-surgery, or have been placed in a skilled nursing unit after having lived in the same home for 30 years. The individual may be cognitively aware, or part of the trauma may be intensified by confusion, delirium, or pain (see Table 2.1). In nursing, we are taught that caring and empathy are valued in our patient interactions. But if we don't strategize to sustain and restore our psyches and souls, we are just as vulnerable as our patients.

TABLE 2.1 NURSING CLINICAL SETTINGS AND EXAMPLES OF EXPOSURE TO TRAUMA

NURSING SETTING	NURSING EXPOSURE TO PATIENT TRAUMAS
Acute care	Emergency and urgent situations where patients feel vulnerable and in crises. Unexpected diagnostic information. Visual, auditory, tactile, and olfactory scenes of intense physical and emotional distress.
Home care	Witnessing adults and children in unsafe environments. Exposure to poverty and food insecurity.
Long-term care	Grief processes that are complicated by cognitive and other impairments. Seeing staff objectify older adults.
Community/Public health	Group events that appear unsafe or in geographic locations that have high crime rates. Post-disaster efforts with multiple traumas impacting individuals on a large scale.
Primary care	Agitated patients or those seeking substances that are contra-indicated. Patients lacking the resources necessary to carry out treatment plan (for example, lack of or insufficient insurance).
Education: School nursing	Seeing others being bullied by peers or faculty. Witnessing patients' pain and suffering for the first time in different clinical areas.

As Table 2.1 illustrates, several areas of clinical practice bring us into the worlds of patients who carry with them the pain of trauma.

TRAUMA-INFORMED REFLECTION

Experiencing trauma through listening and offering comfort can be exhausting. Yet, that comfort, when offered at the appropriate time, can support patients and their families in healing. How will you ensure a balance of empathetic listening and caring efforts, while protecting your own sense of well-being to avoid compassion fatigue?

HISTORICAL TRAUMA

The concept of historical trauma began in 2001 with Kellermann's seminal work that examined Holocaust survivors' traumatic experiences and the transmission of the effects of those experiences to their children and grandchildren. In this paper as well as previous work, Kellermann (2001) attempts to address the question of how trauma is transmitted from one generation to the subsequent generation.

Intergenerational trauma, then, is the nexus of historical trauma in many respects. The lack of resolution, healing, and processing of traumatic events leaves subsequent generations vulnerable to the effects of the original traumatic stress. This became apparent when Karen was performing a pilot intervention study with rural-dwelling kinship parents (Foli, Kersey, Zhang, Woodcox, & Wilkinson, 2018; Foli, Woodcox, Kersey, & Zhang, 2018). These kinship parents, often grandparents, had assumed the care of their grandchildren, who had been removed from their birthparents' care. Mental health services were scarce, and there had been a significant upsurge in the number of children locally and nationally who had been placed in either foster or relative care due to the opioid crisis. Many of the parents had become dependent upon and misused substances and unable to care for their children and provide a safe environment for them.

With extension educators (field-based lay educators), Karen's team implemented a trauma-informed parenting class in rural counties in Indiana. The curriculum, designed by the National Child Traumatic Stress Network (NCTSN; Grillo, Lott, & Foster Care Subcommittee of the Child Welfare Committee, National Child Traumatic Stress Network, 2010), was specific for resource parents, which includes adoptive, foster, and kinship parents. The lessons offered expertly crafted information, ranging from the biological changes a child's brain undergoes when faced with trauma to the often-challenging behaviors that were born from such events. The last module describes secondary trauma that kinship parents can experience when learning of the child's past trauma and pain.

The team and families would meet in safe places, such as the YMCA and county libraries. The children were engaged in play activities with nursing students, so the kinship parents could be attentive to the trauma-informed information. The grandparents would often sit down and freely express what they were experiencing, eager to share with others. Some described their grandchildren's behaviors they simply weren't prepared to address: sexual acting out, aggression, nightmares, and hoarding of food. Some shared guilt over their parenting skills and blamed themselves for their sons' and daughters' faults, which they attributed to the child being removed from the home. Still others confessed to their own traumatic events.

Karen had arrived early to the last class to assist with the setup, and just prior to beginning, one older grandmother sat down next to her. Karen turned to her and offered a smile of welcome. She met Karen's eyes and said in a whispered voice, "I was abused when I was a child. I never told anyone that." Karen saw such a mixture of emotions in her eyes and body language. First there was relief at speaking her secret, the unspeakable, to another human being. Karen met her eyes and nodded slightly, trying to convey acceptance and comfort. The woman then paused, hesitant. Karen interpreted this to signify the fear of risking such a disclosure. The older woman also seemed surprised—but pleased—that she had shared such an intimate experience. About that time, more people situated themselves close by, and the conversation ended. Karen tried to meet her eyes again, and fleetingly did so. Due to the activity for the rest of the day, Karen was unable to follow up with her. But the interaction reminded Karen of intergenerational trauma, the secrets kept for decades, and the invisible yet real posttraumatic influences that may be passed down from generation to generation, often without the person being aware of these effects.

Historical trauma is also an influence for many African Americans. In a position statement by the NCTSN (2016), the following was asserted:

> In spite of progress, the legacy of slavery has been carried forward in many areas of American society, including the racially related injustices that persist, such as mass incarceration, and the lethal violence directed disproportionately toward African Americans. As such, the impact of the unresolved historical trauma of slavery on intergenerational trauma and community trauma should be addressed within a child trauma services framework. Embedded institutional racism associated with these traumas is not yet adequately addressed in child trauma care and continues to shape current policies and attitudes. (para. 2)

Our politics shape our view of trauma. With insight into psychological trauma, we can increase our understanding of views of self, others, and society in a way that can increase our own competencies as caregiver. For example, we have a child of color whom we adopted as an infant. Looking back, our naivete regarding race relations in the US is a compelling case study. As her parents, our daughter's skin color was inconsequential to us. But what we didn't realize is that our perspective was only one piece of her experiences. Through interactions with the adoption community, we realized she wouldn't have the luxury of being colorblind and would need to be able to face the realities of a different world.

TRAUMA-INFORMED REFLECTION

Think about your parents and grandparents. What traumatic events have they faced in their lives? Perhaps they lived through World War II, the Vietnam War, or the Great Depression. If part of your heritage, how has slavery impacted your view of life and society? Does your family discuss related experiences with you as they share their narratives? How have their lives/your life been affected by such intergenerational events?

NURSES AS AN OPPRESSED GROUP

Some might argue that nurses have historically been an oppressed group. Perhaps our oppression has been a function of gender, perhaps our humble roots as unpaid caregivers in the home, and perhaps because nurses are viewed as a significant (group/de-personified) expense on the balance sheets of healthcare organizations. Our expense or budget liability stands in contrast to the medical-industrial complex that profited from individual medical providers. Our voices have been, on certain occasions, muffled, silenced, and censored. In a concept analysis of oppression and its relationship to nursing, Dong and Temple (2011) cited three attributes: 1) unjust treatment; 2) the denial of rights; and 3) the dehumanizing of individuals (p. 172). The authors conclude that nurses are both an oppressed group and, in turn, work with oppressed groups (Dong & Temple, 2011).

With a focus on trauma, horizontal violence or incivility in the workplace—and the psychological injuries that result—may be explained by nurses as an oppressed group. In *Pedagogy of the Oppressed* (1971), Paulo Freire forwards a theory of how oppressed individuals are silenced when confronted with those in authority. Fear, low self-esteem, and marginalization result. Then these emotions give way to anger and aggression toward their own group members. In this case, it is violence from one nurse to another. These behaviors, if Freire is correct, set us up within the profession to propagate our own historical trauma.

Roberts, DeMarco, and Griffin (2009) were one of the first groups of scholars to link such oppressed behaviors to the culture of nursing. More recently, Croft and Cash (2012) situate oppression within the organization (a hegemonic/dominant force) that significantly impacts nurses' lived experiences within institutions. Specifically, four prisms of understanding horizontal/lateral violence through discourse are named: economy and workload (causative factor due to economics of nurses' work); lack of interpersonal skills (blaming the nurse and keeping them marginalized); lack of management skills (managers based on seniority who themselves are isolated); and hierarchical and generational factors (organizational structures and practices; Croft & Cash, 2012). The questions become: Do we continually treat our new nurses as objects, and therefore, treat them in ways that ignore their rights as human beings and colleagues? And if we do, do these abhorrent behaviors stem from being oppressed?

TREATMENT TRAUMA

Nurses frequently see a full spectrum of individuals in need of care, from health promotion and prevention practices to those who are critically ill and injured. Recently, the healthcare context has been viewed as a source of trauma to those who have faced critical illnesses and cancer treatment. We believe this to be especially true with two patient groups who have undergone invasive, pain-inducing, and complex treatment: those who have been patients in the intensive care unit and those who are cancer survivors.

The *Diagnostic and Statistical Manual of Mental Disorders*, Fifth Edition (DSM-5; American Psychiatric Association [APA], 2013), describes a diagnosis of cancer as a traumatic event only when it is sudden and seen as catastrophic. However, based on the *Diagnostic and Statistical Manual of Mental Disorders,* Fourth Edition (DSM-4; APA, 1994), a diagnosis of cancer was included with other serious illnesses and viewed as a potentially traumatic stressor. Using the DSM-4 (APA, 1994) description, researchers who conducted a meta-analysis reported that cancer survivors are 1.66 times more likely to experience PTSD than individuals who had not been diagnosed with cancer (Swartzman, Booth, Munro, & Sani, 2017). In a slightly earlier study, risk factors for cancer-related PTSD were those who were younger in age, had been diagnosed with more advanced stages of cancer, and had completed treatment recently (Abbey, Thompson, Hickish, & Heathcote, 2015). Further evidence of the presence and impact of PTSS, however, was found by James, Harris, Kronish, Wisnivesky, and Lin (2018). These researchers describe early cancer survivors' adherence to self-management of diabetes mellitus being negatively impacted by the presence of PTSS.

Increasingly, cancer is being viewed as a chronic illness. This chronicity brings the potential for recurrence and cycles of treatment. For the cancer survivor, these memories may bring trauma triggers of past psychological and physical pain. In a concept analysis of survivor in the cancer context (Hebdon, Foli, & McComb, 2015), the authors describe how individuals who have survived cancer have been impacted in positive and negative ways. Follow-up screenings, long-term side effects from treatment, and the memories from receiving painful treatments are cited in this concept analysis and set cancer apart from other illnesses for survivors of the disease. In the "Cancer Survivor's Treatment Trauma" sidebar, we present a narrative about the family impact of a cancer diagnosis.

CANCER SURVIVOR'S TREATMENT TRAUMA

Paul was an active pricing analyst in his late fifties. Married later in life, he and his wife, Beth, had two children in elementary and middle schools. As the sole source of income, he knew his family depended upon him. Despite increasing pain in his left side, he continued to work full time until the pain prevented him from eating. Paul surmised that the discomfort was probably due to a problem with his gall bladder—his mother had hers removed at about the same age. However, over the past two days, his pain tolerance was exceeded, and he decided that Beth should drive him to the ED.

Upon arrival, his blood pressure was noted to be 180/92 with a heart rate of 110 beats per minute. Oxygen saturation was 95%. After a detailed history and presenting problem assessment were done, the physician ordered a CT scan of the abdomen as well as other baseline laboratory tests to rule out myocardial infarction, among other emergent issues.

The test results stunned Paul and his wife. A large mass was found, extending from his spleen to his pancreas. Pancreatic cancer was a strong possibility; however, without a tissue biopsy, the diagnosis could not be confirmed. Both he and Beth knew what such a diagnosis would mean.

Within an hour, Paul was in an ambulance, on intravenous morphine sulfate, headed to a large urban medical center an hour and a half from home. His life changed within the span of three hours, from thinking that he needed a cholecystectomy to wondering whether his life would continue and, if it did, what that would look like for him and his family.

The next two weeks were filled with uncertainty and painful procedures for Paul and bureaucracy, worry, and psychological pain for Beth. The good news was that the biopsy had confirmed a treatable cancer: stage III diffuse large B-cell (DLBC), non-Hodgkin lymphoma. The treatment, R-CHOP (rituximab, cyclophosphamide, doxorubicin hydrochloride, vincristine sulfate, and prednisone), carried multiple side effects, including thrombocytopenia, fatigue, fever, anorexia, and immunosuppression. During a short surgical procedure, a port was placed under Paul's skin in his right shoulder area to prevent tissue damage from chemotherapy that may occur in a peripheral IV. Insurance forms, short-term disability, and communications with Paul's company filled Beth's days as she tried to determine how they would financially survive.

Over the next 18 months, the family supported Paul during his treatment: six cycles of R-CHOP. Paul's personality changed every time he took the prednisone to prepare for the chemotherapy agents. Irritability, hyperactivity, and lack of sleep were uncharacteristic of him and created tension at home. When off the prednisone, he was lethargic, sitting in a chair for hours at a time and tasting metal from the chemotherapy agents. He lost his hair, and Beth had to shave the wisps that remained from his head.

Beth took a part-time job to fill in financially where the short-term disability payments fell short. The children pitched in more at home and made sure Paul was taken care of when Beth was working. Slowly, Paul improved, and although still receiving chemotherapy, follow-up tests at seven months post diagnosis confirmed that his cancer was in remission.

However, the good news, while joyously received by Paul, Beth, and their children, wasn't the end of their journey. Paul, in particular, feared a recurrence, unsure whether he could endure additional cycles of R-CHOP. Every six months, he dreaded the repeat scan and follow-up visit with his oncologist to determine whether the cancer was back in his body. He became hypervigilant about his health, experienced recurrent nightmares of painful procedures, and visited his primary care physician for minor concerns. Though he returned to work, he had difficulty concentrating, and his hearing had been affected due to the cancer treatment.

Beth, sensing Paul's increasing stress and what appeared to be reactions to past traumatic experiences, arranged for him to become involved in a cancer survivor support group offered through their local hospital. Paul resisted the support group initially, believing it was a private experience and not one he wanted to relive with strangers. However, at Beth's insistence, he began attending. After several months, Paul began to be more relaxed and optimistic about the future, planning realistic physical activity and consuming an improved diet. His quality of sleep improved, and he became more engaged with the children and Beth. With time, Paul also began to feel a sense of safety and spiritual growth, knowing that whatever may happen in the future, he had supportive people in his life. He felt empowered with knowledge from past experiences and confident that he and his family had survived and could do so again.

Paul's story ended well with physical remission from cancer and psychological growth post trauma. Feeling less isolated as he connected to others who shared a similar narrative and coming to the realization that he could define safety in a new way were components of his psychological recovery.

Treatment trauma is not a new phenomenon. One of the most profound works of literature is the semi-autobiographical novel *Cancer Ward*, by Aleksandr Solzhenitsyn (1969). In this work, Solzhenitsyn details life in a cancer ward in the Soviet Union in 1955, two years following Stalin's death. The physicians, nurses, and patients experience life and healthcare under brutal and stark conditions. The central question Solzhenitsyn poses is: What is the price of being cured? The protagonist, a 34-year-old former army sergeant, Kostoglotov, pleads with the physician whom he begged for treatment:

> And therefore you make the logical deduction that I am to you to be saved at any price! But I don't want to be saved at any price! There isn't anything in the world for which I'd agree to pay any price! (p. 75)

Has our approach changed so much since the time of *Cancer Ward*? What is the price each of us is willing to figuratively pay to be treated, to be saved from illness? Do we ask our patients what the price is for them? These are ethical questions with economic ramifications that our healthcare system leaders cannot seem to completely answer. Kostoglotov continues to discuss suffering and alleviation of suffering. And with the pain and suffering relieved, he begs to "Only now, let me go" (p. 75). One thinks of palliative care and our system of prolonging life based on odds ratios and available treatment. We have spoken to healthcare providers who experience secondary trauma because of what they perceive to be prolonged suffering and the "price of being cured."

TRAUMA WITHIN THE ORGANIZATION AND THE PROFESSIONAL ROLE OF BEING A NURSE

In our professional capacities and roles, we are actors in traumatic events. In this section, we describe how, through our interactions with patients in different ways and contexts, we are exposed to, directly experience, and even create traumatic events. Due to human error, we may be culpable of injuries caused by nursing errors, leaving us and our patients with traumatic stress. Conversely, our lives can change as quickly as a flash of lightning: As caregivers, we may be suddenly assaulted by patients, or as humanitarians and first responders, we experience and witness human suffering in the aftermath of disasters. Remembering the intricacies of our roles allows us to act in safe ways to protect ourselves and our patients.

PATIENT SAFETY AND SECOND-VICTIM TRAUMA

Imagine you're in a clinical experience with your nursing instructor, and it is the first day to "pass meds" in a long-term care facility that still uses paper records. The instructor is distracted and called out of the room. But first, she tells you to get everything ready for her inspection. In the interim, a staff nurse comes into the crowded "med room," and your process is disrupted when she needs to check the med sheets to administer a pain medication. When you return to the records, you are careful to resume the retrieval of meds from the drawer and compare them to the order sheet. The instructor arrives, verifies the meds, and instructs you to go ahead and administer them to the patient, which you do. You return to document your actions and realize you have given a diuretic at the wrong time, doubling the prescribed dose. Your heart pounds as you look for your instructor to tell her. You wonder whether the patient will be harmed by what you did. You also wonder what will happen to your grade.

Approximately 20 years ago, the Institute of Medicine (2000) published a report that changed the way medical errors in US healthcare were perceived. The report described the startling prevalence of patient deaths per year due to medical errors. More than that, the report led the way to make safety a priority in discussions surrounding healthcare. Additional disciplines, such as engineering, were brought into conversations to broaden the perspective from individual culpability to system failures. Organizations brought forth concerted industry efforts to provide safer care. Two examples are the Institute for Healthcare Improvement, which was founded in 1991, and the Agency for Healthcare Research and Quality (2018), which is the lead federal agency charged with improving patient safety.

As increasing attention has been paid to patient safety and quality improvement efforts, so, too has our focus changed to how system defects, provider workarounds (improvisations in care delivery that often deviate from accepted procedures; Debono et al., 2013), and other organizational factors can negatively impact safety. Think of the crowded med room and the interruptions that may have led to the error described at the beginning of this section.

But as our ability to see, and often address, such factors has improved the patient experience, we now realize there is a second victim: the provider who made the error (Wu, 2000). Since that time, several approaches to supporting the second victim have been implemented in various healthcare organizations. How does trauma factor into this second-victim phenomenon? Scott and colleagues (2010) defined the second victim as a:

> Health care provider involved in an unanticipated adverse patient event, medical error and/or a patient-related injury who becomes victimized in the sense that the provider is traumatized by the event. (p. 233)

Second-victim trauma is real and can seriously affect the individual who has made the error. In the helping professions, such as nursing, our motivation often comes from the idea of supporting people and improving their lives and health. To "do harm" via errors is difficult to process. Such errors can lead to serious outcomes, including long-term disability and even death.

Most of the work that has examined second-victim trauma has been located in the acute care setting with bedside clinicians. We review the ways that organizations are stepping up to support nurses who have made errors in the delivery of care in Chapter 5. For now, you should be aware that advanced practice nurses also experience trauma when medical errors are made. Delacroix (2017) describes the impact of medical errors with nurse practitioners through a phenomenological (qualitative) study. The author describes how the nurses experience a "yearning for forgiveness and a supportive other" (p. 403).

WORKPLACE VIOLENCE

In much of the literature, incivility, bullying, lateral, and horizontal violence are subsumed in the category of workplace violence. We discussed this phenomenon in the earlier "Nurses as an Oppressed Group" section. For our purposes here, we examine verbal and physical abuse from patients and visitors directed toward nurses. With the ability to use phones to capture real-time events, almost everyone is a cameraperson. These images have found their ways into social media, journalists' accounts, and in society. For nurses, videos document the extent of workplace violence that healthcare providers encounter. According to the American Nurses Association (ANA; 2018), one in four nurses has been assaulted in the workplace. This troubling statistic raises concerns at both an individual and an organizational level and on a global scale (Wei, Chiou, Chien, & Huang, 2016; Zhang et al., 2017). In the US, a movement is underway to "end nurse abuse" (ANA, 2018). These incidents counter our notions of patient behaviors, as patients are often assumed to be grateful and passive recipients of our benevolent care. The US Department of Labor (n.d.) defines workplace violence as:

> An action (verbal, written, or physical aggression) which is intended to control or cause, or is capable of causing, death or serious bodily injury to oneself or others, or damage to property. Workplace violence includes abusive behavior toward authority, intimidating or harassing behavior, and threats. (n.p.)

In terms of trauma, both physical and psychological damage may result. Our feelings of safety have been shattered because we wonder whom we can trust as we render care. Certain physical spaces carry more risk, such as EDs. In one study, Speroni, Fitch, Dawson, Dugan, and Atherton (2014) reported that out of 762 nurses, 76% experienced workplace violence (physical or verbal abuse by patients or visitors). White male patients ages 26 to 35 years were the most cited group to inflict harm and were often under the influence of alcohol or other substances, or confused (Speroni et al., 2014).

In April 2018, the Joint Commission issued Sentinel Event 59: Physical and Verbal Violence Against Healthcare Workers. In 1996, the Joint

Commission released a sentinel event policy, which defined these serious events as not necessarily related to the patient's condition and those needing immediate attention and response. In Sentinel Event 59, the Joint Commission (2018) described what constitutes workplace violence: the everyday occurrences directed toward those who work in healthcare, from name calling to choking, spitting, and punching. As a way of providing guidance to healthcare organizations, the Joint Commission recommended seven actions. (See the sidebar "The Joint Commission: Sentinel Event on Workplace Violence.") In addition to those listed, nurses need to report the incidents in question to their supervisors, security staff, and even law enforcement. Unfortunately, nurses often do not report incidents of violence. Nurses often excuse such behaviors and rationalize them in various ways:

- The patient didn't know what he was doing (for example, due to dementia, mental illness, extreme emotional state, etc.).

- There was no permanent injury sustained.

- Everyone is bullied. Name calling and so on are inherent in nursing.

- I've seen my coworkers endure this type of behavior.

- I'm careful, but this was probably my fault. I was in a hurry and didn't assess the situation well enough. I put myself in harm's way.

- What are they (such as nurse managers, risk managers, chief nursing officers) going to do about it? There's nothing they can do.

- It was a unique situation. There's no need to make a big deal out of it.

- I don't want anyone to be punished or investigated.

- I don't have time to report it, and I surely don't have enough time to be part of an investigation.

- What if I'm blamed or something goes in my file? I don't want to be labeled as a troublemaker or weak.

- I just want to put it behind me and forget it.

- I'm leaving the organization anyway, so it doesn't make any difference whether I report it.

By labeling workplace violence as a sentinel event, we can understand the importance of these occurrences. Nurses should remind themselves that by reporting situations, they may be helping to identify system issues that can be addressed, moving beyond the individual level to an organization and policy level. Think about those nurses whom you work with. By reporting workplace violence, we support defining and describing the extent and frequency of such violence. Additionally, by reporting incidents, we contribute to the solutions that can be found and, thereby, contribute to supporting a safer environment for both patients and our peers.

As importantly, we've discussed healing from trauma. Workplace violence has both a physical and a psychological component. We believe the psychological trauma occurs most frequently, if not in all cases. By not reporting or sharing the incident with those who can effect change at the system level, paradoxically, nurses deny themselves an opportunity to heal at an individual level. It may become something unspeakable and lay buried within the nurse, shut off from the opportunity to heal the wound that has been inflicted. By remaining silent, we do a disservice to ourselves, our peers, and our organization and create limitations for providing safety in our environments.

TRAUMA-INFORMED REFLECTION

Suppose your co-student and friend has been grabbed in a sexually inappropriate manner by a patient during a medical/surgical clinical experience. (Her breast was squeezed while checking an IV line.) Your friend was assertive and instructed the patient to stop touching her. The patient immediately apologized, stating it must have been the medications he's taking that contributed to his inappropriate behavior. Your friend is adamant about not reporting the event but is shaken and confused. What would you say to her? What is the priority for your friend? For the student's faculty instructor and the school? For the healthcare organization?

THE JOINT COMMISSION: SENTINEL EVENT ON WORKPLACE VIOLENCE

The Joint Commission's suggested seven actions:

- Clearly define workplace violence and put systems in place across the organization that enable staff to report workplace violence instances, including verbal abuse.

- Recognizing that data come from several sources, capture, track and trend all reports of workplace violence—including verbal abuse and attempted assaults when no harm occurred.

- Provide appropriate follow-up and support to victims, witnesses, and others affected by workplace violence, including psychological counseling and trauma-informed care if necessary.

- Review each case of workplace violence to determine contributing factors. Analyze data related to workplace violence, and worksite conditions, to determine priority situations for interventions.

- Develop quality improvement initiatives to reduce incidents of workplace violence.

- Train all staff, including security, in de-escalation, self-defense, and response to emergency codes.

- Evaluate workplace violence reduction initiatives.

© *The Joint Commission, 2018. Reprinted with permission.*

NURSING AND SUICIDE

Knowing someone who has attempted or committed suicide increases most nurses' psychological discomfort. What is perhaps more disconcerting is when a nurse chooses to end her life. Increasing attention has been focused on nurse suicide with a noted lack of available data (Davidson, Mendis, Stuck, DeMichele, & Zisook, 2018). In the US, we are still searching for definitive trends and answers to why nurses choose to end their lives. However, in England, recent statistics point to a troubling finding: Between 2011 and 2015, nurse suicides were 23% above the national average (Windsor-Shellard, 2017). Zeng, Zhou, Yan, Yang, and Jin (2018) studied suicide rates of nurses in China by reviewing public reports. Findings include 46 nurse deaths by suicide; 98% were female, and the most common way was by jumping off a building. They reported data were scarce, but that, "Overall, Chinese nurses work under too much pressure, overwork, depression, suicide and other things together broke their white angel wings" ("Introduction," para. 4). Suppositions related to nurse suicides are exposure to medications and knowledge of methods of ending one's life; occupational stress; giving to others without giving to self; high-stress environments, from acute care to home health; and incivility-embedded organizations.

We believe concentrating on the traumatic aspects of these factors may lead to opening the conversations around the sad journeys of nurses electing to end their lives. Evidence supports the relationship between trauma and suicide. Could such an approach allow us to ask the right questions at the right time to intervene and avoid such loss? The dichotomy of "white angel wings" and the brutality of what nurses are often exposed to leads us to wonder whether being mindful of the effects of trauma could be a place to begin.

TRAUMA SURROUNDING DISASTERS

As with other first responders and subsequent caregivers, nurses face traumatic stress during disasters, from ministering to others to experiencing firsthand the effects of disasters. Since 9/11, with the four coordinated terrorist attacks against the US, we have been on alert for man-made disasters. Yet the term "disaster" is complex, with several descriptions possible (for example, natural versus man-made and acute versus long-term impact). The United Nations Office for Disaster Risk Reduction (2017) defines disaster as:

> A serious disruption of the functioning of a community or a
> society at any scale due to hazardous events interacting with
> conditions of exposure, vulnerability and capacity, leading to
> one or more of the following: human, material, economic and
> environmental losses and impacts. Annotations: The effect of

the disaster can be immediate and localized, but is often wide-spread and could last for a long period of time. The effect may test or exceed the capacity of a community or society to cope using its own resources, and therefore may require assistance from external sources, which could include neighbouring jurisdictions, or those at the national or international levels. ("Disaster," para. 1–2)

From this description, we understand the fluidity of the scope and scales of disasters and, therefore, the impact on resources. Disasters may be created by large masses, such as shifts in tectonic plates, or microorganisms, such as those causing infectious diseases. Disaster relief efforts may be made within a structure, such as a hospital, or in the open environment/community, at temporary shelters. As the largest workforce of healthcare professionals, nurses have been, are, and will be drawn into disaster relief efforts. Although their work was preliminary in nature, Baack and Alfred (2013) found that most of their sample of 620 rural-based nurses did not feel confident in responding to disasters; those with previous experiences with disasters felt the most confident. The ANA (2017) challenges nurses to become prepared. For a historical perspective on nurses and their role in disasters, both natural and man-made, see Wall and Keeling (2010).

The ANA (2017) has issued a policy statement on nurses' role in disasters. The ANA, while acknowledging the ethical imperative of the nurse's response, also describes legal and regulatory issues as well as safety, including ongoing violence. In the 2017 document, the ANA also describes secondary trauma by citing possible situations in which the nurse would have to "walk past a mortally wounded person to treat someone else, or to take a terminally ill patient off a ventilator to allocate it to a patient with a better chance of survival" (p. 3). Such dilemmas have the potential to become traumatic events that create lasting psychological harm for the nurse.

CONCLUSIONS

Chapter 2 describes those unique traumas and traumatic events that nurses experience. We included secondary trauma, compassion fatigue, historical trauma, nurses as an oppressed group, trauma experienced because of the treatment offered in the healthcare system, second-victim trauma/trauma resulting from errors, workplace violence, nurse suicide, and trauma surrounding disasters. For students and new nurses, it is important to understand the ways in which trauma may be experienced because of their professional responsibilities.

HIGHLIGHTS OF CHAPTER CONTENT

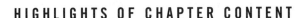

- Nurses are particularly susceptible to secondary trauma and compassion fatigue due to the nature of their work. Examples are offered based on the setting where care is offered.

- Historical and intergenerational trauma may be difficult to assess; however, the nurse should be aware of its impact on patients.

- When viewed as an oppressed group, the actions of the nurse may explain the horizontal violence seen in the workplace and academia.

- Nurses should be aware of the potential of causing trauma to patients while administering treatment plans.

- Medical errors not only cause patient safety issues but also have the potential of causing second-victim trauma for the nurse.

- Workplace violence is increasing and creates significant physical and psychological trauma; the Joint Commission (2018) has classified workplace violence as a sentinel event.

- Disasters may be sources of professionally related traumas, including secondary trauma, fears related to physical safety, and a lack of preparedness.

REFERENCES

Abbey, G., Thompson, S. B. N., Hickish, T., & Heathcote, D. (2015). A meta-analysis of prevalence rates and moderating factors for cancer-related post-traumatic stress disorder. *Psycho-Oncology, 24*, 371–381. doi:10.1002/pon.3654

Agency for Healthcare Research and Quality. (2018). A profile. Retrieved from http://www.ahrq.gov/cpi/about/profile/index.html

American Nurses Association. (2017). *Who will be there? Ethics, the law, and a nurse's duty to respond in a disaster* (Issue brief). Retrieved from https://www.nursingworld.org/~4ad845/globalassets/docs/ana/who-will-be-there_disaster-preparedness_2017.pdf

American Nurses Association. (2018). #EndNurseAbuse: Take the pledge. Retrieved from http://p2a.co/t84cVfR

American Psychiatric Association. (1994). *Diagnostic and statistical manual of mental disorders* (4th ed.). Washington, DC: Author.

American Psychiatric Association. (2013). *Diagnostic and statistical manual of mental disorders* (5th ed.). Arlington, VA: Author.

Baack, S., & Alfred, D. (2013). Nurses' preparedness and perceived competence in managing disasters. *Journal of Nursing Scholarship, 45*(3), 281–287. doi:10.1111/jnu.12029

Coetzee, S. K., & Klopper, H. C. (2010). Compassion fatigue in nursing practice: A concept analysis. *Nursing and Health Sciences, 12*, 235–243. doi:10.1111/j.1442-2018.2010.00526.x

Croft, R. K., & Cash, P. A. (2012). Deconstructing contributing factors to bullying and lateral violence in nursing using a postcolonial feminist lens. *Contemporary Nurse, 42*(2), 226–242. doi:10.5172/conu.2012.42.2.226

Davidson, J., Mendis, J., Stuck, A. R., DeMichele, G., & Zisook, S. (2018). *Nurse suicide: Breaking the silence*. Discussion paper, National Academy of Medicine, Washington, DC. Retrieved from https://nam.edu/nurse-suicide-breaking-the-silence

Debono, D. S., Greenfield, D., Travaglia, J. F., Long, J. C., Black, D., Johnson, J., & Braithwaite, J. (2013). Nurses' workarounds in acute healthcare settings: A scoping review. *BMC Health Services Research, 13*, 175. doi:10.1186/1472-6963-13-175

Delacroix, R. (2017). Exploring the experience of nurse practitioners who have committed medical errors: A phenomenological approach. *Journal of the American Association of Nurse Practitioners, 29*, 403–409. doi:10.1002/2327-6924.12468

Dong, D., & Temple, B. (2011). Oppression: A concept analysis and implications for nurses and nursing. *Nursing Forum, 46*(3), 169–176.

Foli, K. J., Kersey, S., Zhang, L., Woodcox, S., & Wilkinson, B. (2018). Trauma-informed parenting classes delivered to rural kinship parents: A pilot study. *The Journal of the American Psychiatric Nurses Association, 24*(1), 62–75. doi:10.1177/1078390317730605

Foli, K. J., Woodcox, S., Kersey, S., & Zhang, L. (2018). Addressing the wicked problem of childhood trauma through a nursing and cooperative extension system collaboration. *Public Health Nursing, 35*(1), 56–63. doi:10.1111/phn.12375

Freire, P. (1971). *Pedagogy of the oppressed*. New York, NY: Herder & Herder.

Georges, J. M. (2011). Evidence of the unspeakable: Biopower, compassion, and nursing. *Advances in Nursing Science, 34*(2), 130–135. doi:10.1097/ANS.0b013e31826cd8

Grillo, C. A., Lott, D. A., & Foster Care Subcommittee of the Child Welfare Committee, National Child Traumatic Stress Network. (2010). *Caring for children who have experienced trauma: A workshop for resource parents—Facilitator's guide*. Los Angeles, CA, & Durham, NC: National Child Traumatic Stress Network.

Hebdon, M., Foli, K., & McComb, S. (2015). Survivor in the cancer context: A concept analysis. *Journal of Advanced Nursing, 71*(8), 1774–1786. doi:10.1111/ jan.12646

Institute of Medicine. (2000). *To err is human: Building a safer health system.* Washington, DC: The National Academies Press. doi:https://doi.org/10.17226/9728

James, J., Harris, Y. T., Kronish, I. M., Wisnivesky, J. P., & Lin, J. J. (2018). Exploratory study of impact of cancer-related posttraumatic stress symptoms on diabetes self-management among cancer survivors. *Psycho-Oncology, 27*, 648–653. doi:10.1002/ pon.4568

The Joint Commission. (April 18, 2018). *The Joint Commission issues new sentinel event alert on violence against health care workers during Workplace Violence Awareness Month.* Retrieved from https://www.jointcommission.org/the_joint_commission_issues_new_sentinel_event_alert_on_violence_against_health_care_workers_during_workplace_violence_awareness_month/

Kellermann, N. P. F. (2001). Transmission of Holocaust trauma: An integrative view. *Psychiatry, 64*(3), 256–267. doi:https://doi.org/10.1521/psyc.64.3.256.18464

National Child Traumatic Stress Network. (2016). *Racial injustice and trauma: African Americans in the US* [Position statement]. Retrieved from https://www.nctsn.org/sites/default/files/resources/racial_injustice_and_trauma_african_americans_in_the_us.pdf

Roberts, S. J., DeMarco, R., & Griffin, M. (2009). The effect of oppressed group behaviors on the culture of the nursing workplace: A review of the evidence and interventions for change. *Journal of Nursing Management, 17*(3), 288–293.

Scott, S. D., Hirschinger, L. E., Cox, K. R., McCoig, M., Hahn-Cover, K., Epperly, K. M., . . . Hall, L. W. (2010). Caring for our own: Deploying a systemwide second victim rapid response team. *The Joint Commission Journal on Quality and Patient Safety, 36*(5), 233–240.

Sendelbach, S., & Funk, M. (2013). Alarm fatigue: A patient safety concern. *AACN Advanced Critical Care, 24*(4), 378–386. doi:10.1097/NCI.0b013e3182a903f9

Solzhenitsyn, A. (1969). *Cancer ward.* New York, NY: Farrar, Straus, and Giroux.

Speroni, K. G., Fitch, T., Dawson, E., Dugan, L., & Atherton, M. (2014). Incidence and cost of nurse workplace violence perpetrated by hospital patients or patient visitors. *Journal of Emergency Nursing, 40*(3), 218–228. doi:https://doi.org/10.1016/j.jen.2013.05.014

Substance Abuse and Mental Health Services Administration. (Spring 2014). Key terms: Definitions. *SAMHSA News, 22*(2). Retrieved from https://www.samhsa.gov/samhsaNewsLetter/Volume_22_Number_2/trauma_tip/key_terms.html

Swartzman, S., Booth, J. N., Munro, A., & Sani, F. (2017). Posttraumatic stress disorder after cancer diagnosis in adults: A meta-analysis. *Depression and Anxiety, 34*, 327–339. doi:10.1002/da.22542

United Nations Office for Disaster Risk Reduction. (2017). Terminology. Retrieved from https://www.unisdr.org/we/inform/terminology

US Department of Labor. (n.d.). DOL workplace violence program —Appendices. Retrieved from https://www.dol.gov/oasam/hrc/policies/dol-workplace-violence-program-appendices.htm

Wall, B. M., & Keeling, A. W. (2010). *Nursing on the frontline: When disaster strikes, 1878–2010.* New York, NY: Springer Publishing Company.

Wei, C-Y., Chiou, S-T., Chien, L-Y., & Huang, N. (2016). Workplace violence against nurses—Prevalence and association with hospital organizational characteristics and health-promotion efforts: Cross-sectional study. *International Journal of Nursing Studies, 56*, 63–70. doi:http://dx.doi.org/10.1016/j.ijnurstu.2015.12.012

Windsor-Shellard, B. (March 17, 2017). *Suicide by occupation, England: 2011 to 2015.* Office for National Statistics. Retrieved from https://www.ons.gov.uk/ peoplepopulationandcommunity/birthsdeathsandmarriages/deaths/articles/ suicidebyoccupation/england2011to2015

Wu, A. W. (2000). The second victim: The doctor who makes the mistake needs help too. *BMJ, 320*(7237), 726–727.

Zeng, H. J., Zhou, G. Y., Yan, H. H., Yang, X. H., & Jin, H. M. (2018). Chinese nurses are at high risk for suicide: A review of nurses suicide in China 2007–2016. *Archives of Psychiatric Nursing, 32,* 896–900. doi:https://doi.org/10.1016/j.apnu.2018.07.005

Zhang, L., Wang, A., Xiec, X., Zhouc, Y., Lid, J., Yange, L., & Zhang, J. (2017). Workplace violence against nurses: A cross-sectional study. *International Journal of Nursing Studies, 72,* 8–14. doi:https://doi.org/10.1016/jinurstu.2017.04.002

LEARNING OBJECTIVES

At the end of this chapter, you will be able to:

- Translate the Substance Abuse and Mental Health Services Administration's (SAMHSA, 2014) three E's of trauma for individuals who have experienced trauma.

- Describe the items included in adverse childhood experiences (ACEs) and their prevalence (Felitti et al., 1998) according to the Centers for Disease Control and Prevention (CDC).

- Understand basic approaches to nursing assessments of past trauma in children, adults, and older adults.

- Differentiate between trauma triggers and intrusion symptoms.

- Assess your personal compassion fatigue via the Secondary Traumatic Stress Scale (STSS; Bride, Robinson, & Yegidis, 2004).

- Analyze sources of personal implicit biases that may affect patient care.

ASSESSING FOR PSYCHOLOGICAL TRAUMA

3

PURPOSE OF THE CHAPTER

In this chapter, assessing for past and current trauma will be emphasized. We now turn to how we can assess such history, as well as current
life events, which pose the potential to become stress-inducing and
lingering trauma. Mental health professionals have a ready arsenal of
testing to be performed on individuals to determine whether trauma has
occurred or is occurring. Although we include several ways to interpret
how an individual has been affected by trauma, these are, in general,
not meant to make diagnostic evaluations. In other words, these tests are
not intended to make definitive judgments about an individual's mental
health or diagnoses. In the following pages, we focus on how to expand
our own self-awareness through nursing assessments and place this
within the practice of nursing for the patients we serve.

INDIVIDUALIZED ASSESSMENT

The Substance Abuse and Mental Health Services Administration (SAMH-SA, 2014) leads the US's efforts in understanding trauma and characterizes the concept by the three E's of trauma:

- Event is direct exposure to either a traumatic event or witnessing such an event. The Event also includes severe neglect, which impedes healthy development. This definition aligns with the *Diagnostic and Statistical Manual of Mental Disorders*, Fifth Edition (DSM-5; American Psychiatric Association [APA], 2013) criterion.

- Experience is an individualized encounter. For the Experience to be traumatic, there needs to be a power differential and a search for sense-making ("why me?"). Dependent upon a number of factors, such as cultural beliefs, the chronicity of the trauma, the person inflicting the trauma, and the timing of the trauma in development, the individual will perceive the Event in a unique way.

- Effects is a construct that posits how the aftermath of trauma is different for individuals. These may differ in terms of onset, intensity, duration, and area impacted (physical, cognitive, emotional regulation, and so on). These Effects are increasingly being studied from a neurobiological perspective (see the discussion of telomere length in Chapter 1; SAMHSA, 2014). These Effects are similar to or include posttraumatic stress symptoms (PTSS), such as avoidance, emotional dysregulation, and hypervigilance.

For the nurse, the rule for assessing individuals who have experienced trauma is to gather information in a patient-centered, individualized, holistic manner, free from assumptions, coupled with an awareness of the Event, Experience, and Effects of trauma. In this way, as strategies for comfort and caring are articulated and discussed with the individual, intervention modification and refinement become part of the circular plan of care.

Consider two young adults and how their journeys toward healing can be framed by trauma's three E's.

PHIL: HEALING FROM COMPLEX TRAUMA

Phil is a 21-year-old college student who is majoring in nursing. During his older childhood and adolescence, he moved frequently because his father couldn't seem to hold a job. His best memories are when his father did a brief tour in the military, being deployed to the Middle East for about two years. His mother seemed happier, and his younger brother thrived at school and in sports. Phil stepped up and became almost a coparent and enjoyed being a "super brother." But his father eventually returned when Phil was 15 years old, and the family dynamics changed. No longer was Phil seen as a young adult, but "just a kid who didn't seem to matter." He witnessed his father shouting at his mother, calling her names, and accusing her of being unfaithful. These terrible fights often occurred when his father was intoxicated. His father even waved one of his guns around one night, pushing Phil up against a wall. He'd witness his mother's pleas for him to stop, and the next day, his father would seem genuinely sorry. Once he muttered, "Son, you don't know what I've seen." Phil watched as his brother succumbed to drugs, finally leaving home when Phil left for college.

For the past three years, Phil has enjoyed being at college and being enrolled in nursing courses. He dates and stays away from alcohol and drugs. His grades are solid, and he's begun to interview for positions when he graduates in nine months. Lately, though, he feels despondent and wonders if he'll end up like his dad. He hasn't heard from his brother in months, and his parents have decided to divorce. His class in leadership is his favorite, but he struggles with the content in pediatrics, feeling fuzzy and unfocused. His stomach hurts on a regular basis, with temporary relief when he eats. He self-medicates with antacids and water. Recently, he's been going to church with his girlfriend, Reggie, and trying to make sense of his past. The psychiatric mental health class also provides him with insight into what happened to him as an adolescent. He knows that the pediatrics class might be triggering some of the past secrets, but he's learned about the principles of trauma-informed care and makes the link between his past and present. Reggie supports Phil and listens to him as he carefully and sporadically shares his past.

For Phil, the Event was exposure to domestic violence and the life-threatening situation with his father. The complex, intergenerational, chronic, and developmental trauma affected Phil in cognitive, physical, emotional, and psychological ways. The Experience, processed by Phil, is one of context and influenced by the knowledge he's gained through nursing school. His journey toward healing is in process as he utilizes resources, such as social support, as his grief and mourning take place. The Effects of his trauma are multifaceted, and the onset of symptoms was delayed until there were triggers in his environment: his parents' divorce, his upcoming graduation, and the absence of his brother. The change he is facing as he enters the world as an adult will present challenges, but if he can reestablish a sense of safety, continue to mourn, and seek connections with others, he will be on his path to healing from trauma.

SYDNEY: HEALING FROM ACUTE TRAUMA

Sydney, a 21-year-old nursing student, had grown closer to her mom, Carol, ironically, after leaving for college the year before. She'd become more appreciative of what Carol had done for her as a single parent. While it'd just been the two of them, Sydney had pushed Carol to the periphery of her life during adolescence. But it seemed even through the missteps she'd made, Carol's presence was always constant and supportive. During the summer break between Sydney's freshman and sophomore years of college, the two of them had decided to take a road trip through the state and visit flea markets down a stretch of an old state road. Several days into the trip, they wondered how the car would hold all their purchases. Sydney had offered to drive that evening, as it was several miles to the next stop. The other driver, who'd been declared legally intoxicated, hit their car head on, instantly killing Carol. Sydney spent several days in the hospital with a ruptured spleen and other musculoskeletal injuries. She found when she was discharged that she was truly alone. Her guilt overwhelmed her, and she blamed herself for being the one driving and overfilling the car with purchases—did it make a difference in her being able to see the other car? She wished she could somehow undo that night and take back her offer to drive. She would have gladly been the one killed rather than live so alone. Somehow, with the help of an honest and competent attorney, the small estate was closed, the house sold, and the belongings either donated or stored.

When Sydney returned to her nursing studies, she didn't really care about her appearance and avoided her peers. In addition to her grief, flashbacks intruded upon her thoughts at random times throughout the day, portraying the last second before the car hit them: a bright light and her mother screaming. She slept poorly, despite being exhausted by anxiety during the day. She was hypervigilant with her studies, obsessed with doing well to honor her mother. Her clinical group of peers began to see her as odd and not in sync with the rest of them. They started to exclude her from discussions. They'd stop talking when she entered the room for their postclinical debriefing. Their nonverbal behavior was characterized by incivility: rolling eyes when she would offer a comment, moving physically away from her in an exaggerated way, and working together if someone was behind, but excluding her.

At the end of the semester, Sydney was evaluated by her clinical instructor, Dr. Coats, who held a doctor of nursing practice degree and was about the age of Sydney's mother when she passed. Dr. Coats began the conference by communicating how Sydney was barely meeting the clinical course objectives, which was confusing since her test scores were solid. Sydney began to cry and to describe how hard the semester had been, the car accident that had killed her mom, and the group's bullying behaviors. Dr. Coats listened closely and made notes. She let Sydney talk for several minutes, conveyed sympathy, and murmured, "This explains a lot." Dr. Coats promised to address the group's behaviors and recognized how the grief and traumatic event had put Sydney at risk for failing school due to clinical performance. She encouraged Sydney to speak to one of the academic advisors at the school, who could connect her to counseling resources at the university. Before Sydney left the office, Dr. Coats had called the advisor and made an appointment for her.

Sydney expressed the three E's slightly differently than Phil. Her Event was acute trauma, the car accident that resulted in her mother's death and her survivor's guilt. With the traumatic event, she also experienced a grief reaction. The Experience of the trauma, how she made sense of the event, was complicated by her grief. Developmentally, she regressed in self-care and felt inadequate to meet the adult world. Her wishing for a different outcome and the magnitude of her guilt crippled her emotionally. Her vulnerability and weakness were perceived by her peers, who reacted with bullying and incivility. The Effect of her trauma manifested in her hyper-vigilance to obsessive studying for the lecture/tests, which was in contrast to her performance clinically. Yet, it was Sydney's way of remembering her mother with respect. Her feelings of guilt and of being totally alone in the world impacted her cognitive functioning, and the intrusive thoughts of the night of the accident compounded this effect. Because she was willing to trust Dr. Coats with this information and Dr. Coats was a compassionate listener and trauma-informed faculty member, Sydney was connected with services to help her work toward healing.

ASSESSING FOR PAST TRAUMA

It is not uncommon for those who have experienced highly stressful past events to be consciously unaware of this influence on current thoughts and behaviors. The Event could have occurred long ago, when the individuals were infants, children, or adolescents incapable of expressing the experience. Yet, often, our behaviors tell a different story and become a substitute, a sign, a symptom of the harm caused. Perhaps we have difficulty forming trusting relationships. Or we need to have control over our environment or make decisions in an excessive way. Maybe we have a tendency toward using substances to decrease anxiety. Or we have a hard time regulating the emotions we feel and appropriately expressing those to people around us. Sometimes, we shut down and isolate ourselves.

We begin with a discussion of one of the most prevalent and, in our opinion, concerning trends in our society: the increase in childhood traumatic events, a significant public health concern.

ADVERSE CHILDHOOD EXPERIENCES

In Chapter 1, we discussed how adverse childhood experiences (ACEs) impact adults' morbidities and mortality, especially for those with six or more adverse experiences. We also looked at the economic burden on society as a result of these experiences. In this section, we look specifically at what ACEs are and how prevalent they are. A compelling and troubling estimate is that 45% of all children in the US have experienced one or more ACEs (Sacks & Murphey, 2018).

What are ACEs? An individual's exposure to ACEs provides compelling and powerful evidence that helps us to understand how stressful and potentially traumatic experiences endured in childhood may have long-term effects. Between 1995 and 1997, 17,000 members of a health maintenance organization, Kaiser Permanente, underwent routine physical examinations. These individuals were asked questions related to their experiences as children. The results were startling. See Table 3.1 (Felitti et al., 1998).

TABLE 3.1 ORIGINAL CDC/KAISER PERMANENTE ACE TOOL

ABUSE	WHILE YOU WERE GROWING UP, DURING THE FIRST 18 YEARS OF LIFE…[1]
Emotional abuse	A parent, stepparent, or adult living in your home swore at you, insulted you, put you down, or acted in a way that made you afraid that you might be physically hurt.
Physical abuse	A parent, stepparent, or adult living in your home pushed, grabbed, slapped, threw something at, or hit you so hard that you had marks or were injured.
Sexual abuse	An adult, relative, family friend, or stranger who was at least five years older than you touched or fondled your body in a sexual way, made you touch his/her body in a sexual way, or attempted to have any type of sexual intercourse with you.

continues

TABLE 3.1 ORIGINAL CDC/KAISER PERMANENTE ACE TOOL (CONT.)

HOUSEHOLD DYSFUNCTION	WHILE YOU WERE GROWING UP, DURING THE FIRST 18 YEARS OF LIFE...[1]
Mother treated violently	Your mother or stepmother was pushed, grabbed, slapped, had something thrown at her, kicked, bitten, hit with a fist, hit with something hard, repeatedly hit for at least a few minutes, or threatened or hurt by a knife or gun by your father (or stepfather) or mother's boyfriend.
Household substance abuse	A household member was a problem drinker or alcoholic or a household member used street drugs.
Mental illness in household	A household member was depressed or mentally ill or a household member attempted suicide.
Parental separation or divorce	Your parents were ever separated or divorced.
Criminal household member	A household member went to prison.
NEGLECT	WHILE YOU WERE GROWING UP, DURING THE FIRST 18 YEARS OF LIFE...[1]
Emotional neglect	Someone in your family helped you feel important or special, you felt loved, people in your family looked out for each other and felt close to each other, and your family was a source of strength and support.[2]
Physical neglect	There was someone to take care of you, protect you, and take you to the doctor if you needed it,[2] you didn't have enough to eat, your parents were too drunk or too high to take care of you, and you had to wear dirty clothes.

[1] All ACE questions refer to the respondent's first 18 years of life. (See Felitti et al., 1998.)

[2] Items were reverse-scored to reflect the framing of the question.

Scoring: Respondents were considered exposed to the category if they answered "yes" to one or more in a category. Scores ranged from 0 (not exposed to any category) to 10 (exposed to all categories).

So just how common are ACEs? Based on the original data (Felitti et al., 1998), about 12.5% of participants had experienced four or more ACEs (range 0–10; see Figure 3.1). Remember, the effects of ACEs are dose-dependent, with increasing health risks associated with more ACEs. The three most common ACEs assessed were childhood physical abuse (28%), household substance abuse (27%), and parental separation or divorce (23%; Felitti et al., 1998). What was also important to note is that these ACE scores were reported by middle-class Americans, considered to be a low-risk group for childhood trauma. In an updated discussion, Felitti and Anda (2010) describe the significant associations between ACEs and morbidities in adolescence and adulthood, including chronic depression, suicide attempts, alcohol and substance use (including IV drug use), smoking, impaired worker performance, teen sexual behaviors, liver disease, chronic obstructive lung disease, and heart disease. It would seem that individuals who suffer early in life try ways to lessen and avoid their pain and, at times, numb it, which are counter to mental and physical well-being.

Since the first publication of findings from these events (Felitti et al., 1998), over 50 studies have reported the longitudinal impact of those with ACE scores. In summary, 10 major constructs are typically assessed surrounding (Bethell et al., 2017):

- Physical abuse
- Emotional abuse
- Sexual abuse
- Physical neglect
- Emotional neglect
- Parental separation/divorce
- Parental incarceration
- Domestic violence
- Household mental illness/suicide
- Household substance abuse

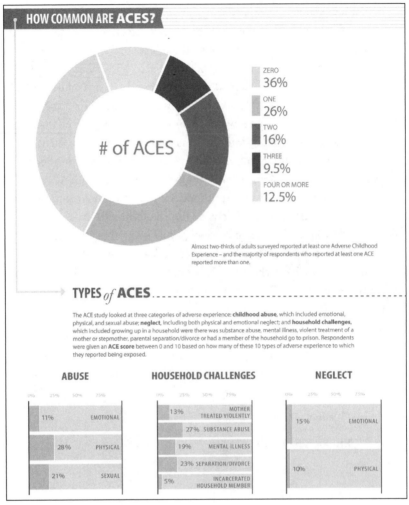

FIGURE 3.1   How common are ACEs?

Source: Centers for Disease Control and Prevention, n.d.

ASSESSMENT: BEHAVIORS ASSOCIATED WITH POSTTRAUMATIC EVENTS

We take a life span approach to describe behaviors that may be influenced by past trauma in children, adolescents, adults, and older adults. The following sections are broad strokes and generalize how individuals may change, depending upon their stage in life, after psychological injury. We know that one of the most prized aspects of nursing is to see our patients, clients, and consumers as individuals with unique narratives and personalities; thus, development is one aspect of assessing for behavioral changes in the aftermath of traumatic events.

CHILDREN AND ADOLESCENTS

Current statistics surrounding childhood trauma present a concerning picture. As of February 2018, nationally, one in ten children have experienced three or more ACEs; in Arizona, Arkansas, Montana, New Mexico, and Ohio, the prevalence rises to one in seven children having experienced three or more ACEs (Sacks & Murphey, 2018). More black, non-Hispanic (61%) and Hispanic (51%) children have experienced at least one ACE when compared with white non-Hispanic (40%) children (Sacks & Murphey, 2018).

Because developmental tasks are accomplished in tandem with brain functioning and the environment, traumatic events manifest with different symptoms based on chronological age. Young children (pre- and young school-aged) may not have the words or the ability to describe what happened to them, contributing to their feelings of helplessness. They may regress in areas that had been mastered, such as toileting, and if the caregiver/parent is unaware of what occurred, the regression may be confusing. Sleep and nighttime routines may be disrupted. Play may focus on the traumatic event or appear to be violent (National Child Traumatic Stress Network [NCTSN], 2010).

Older children may be concerned over their safety and the safety of others. They also may regress on tasks that had previously been achieved. Sleep disturbances and insomnia may also be issues for these children. Feelings may overwhelm them and include guilt, shame, sadness, and perseveration over the event. Others in their environment, such as teachers, may notice difficulty with concentration and distractions. Somatization may also occur, with the child complaining of physical issues related to psychological distress. Last, externalizing behaviors may surface in the form of aggression and striking out toward others (NCTSN, 2010).

Adolescents depend on their peers to achieve a sense of identity. The experience of trauma may contribute to feeling different or abnormal. There may be a shift in how they perceive the world, and this shift may contribute to externalizing behaviors such as high-risk or self-harm. Their anger may result in feelings of revenge or wanting retribution from others (NCTSN, 2010).

Note that because each adult will react in an individual way to traumatic events, the reactions of children and adolescents will also vary. Think of a stew composed of meat, vegetables, and a sauce. The traumatic event, surrounded by the personality and temperament of the person/child, the environment that the person lives in, and the developmental stage yet to be attained will shape the response from the child or adolescent.

Supportive relationships in which attachment has occurred will often buffer the trauma the child or adolescent has experienced. The adult who is able to whisper into the ear of the child in affirming, supportive, and nurturing ways often provides a defense against some of the sequelae caused by trauma (Rahim, 2014). Such relationships, however, may be undermined by the presence of the façade of others' success propagated by social media. Adolescents and young adults have been impacted by social media posts and pictures of perfection. In response, a recently coined term, *Duck Syndrome,* describes young adults, particularly those in college or graduate school, who appear to be content, functioning, and thriving, while below the surface (as a duck would glide on water and thrash underneath), they are struggling with the pressures of daily life (Sun, 2018; see the "Duck Syndrome" sidebar). And not just daily life, but the pressures that accompany the expectations of high performance and success. We encourage you to think about Duck Syndrome for those who have been exposed to trauma and fit into this demographic group. The outward appearance of secure, yet false, success may be especially overwhelming to those who have suffered through traumatic experiences.

DUCK SYNDROME

A student at Stanford University, Sun (2018) coined the term *Duck Syndrome,* which seems to be catching the attention of several parties. Do you believe there is merit in Duck Syndrome? Why do we continually discount that for so many people, there are challenges in life and accept that social media is not a platform for showcasing such a struggle? This negative space—the absence of struggle—becomes filled with fairy tales of individuals who appear to glide on water. Why is telling our stories to those we trust needed?

ADULTS

Based on presenting symptoms, both physical and psychological, thousands of screening, diagnostic, and evaluation procedures and tools exist. For example, screening tools for depression, alcohol and substance use, and PTSD are commonly employed to assess for symptoms of current and past trauma. Although this text isn't designed to provide a comprehensive review of these tools, assessing for past trauma in older children, adolescents, and adults may be straightforward.

Trauma-informed approaches call for a shift in focus from asking individuals, "What's wrong with you?" to instead asking, "What has happened to you?" (SAMHSA-HRSA Center for Integrated Health Solutions, n.d.). The discourse is important because words reflect reality, but also create one. This language sets up the provider to understand the event, injury, or harm rather than erroneously place the burden of explanation of feelings and behaviors on the individual who is in pain. There is another important component to these questions. The first question implies there is something damaged in the individual; there is judgment and condemnation. The second question offers individuals an opportunity to share their narratives in a safe place, with a sense of control, and seek a connection with another. Asking "What has happened to you?" provides acknowledgment and awareness that something has occurred.

TRAUMA TRIGGERS AND INTRUSION SYMPTOMS

A brief distinction between trauma triggers and intrusive thoughts needs to be forwarded. A *trauma trigger* is a stimulus that creates a link to a previous trauma experience. This trigger could be a sound, a scent, or a visual cue of past trauma. For example, a woman experienced psychological abuse in the form of chronic, complex, interpersonal trauma. (Her mother would scream and demean her, which was emotional abuse.) This individual may be shopping at a department store and selecting a perfume. She tests a scent, and the stimulus immediately reminds her of her mother's cologne. This trigger brings back memories of pain and stress from this complex trauma when she was younger, powerless, and shamed.

In contrast, intrusion symptoms are one of the diagnostic criteria for posttraumatic stress disorder (PTSD; APA, 2013). These symptoms are involuntary and distressing; they can take the form of memories, dreams, and flashbacks and include physiological reactions. For children, these intrusions may be communicated through repetitive play (APA, 2013). An example of an intrusion is when a college student has recurrent nightmares about being bullied in high school. His sleep is disrupted by "reliving" name calling, being excluded during lunch, and being threatened after school. He usually awakens with an accelerated heart rate and diaphoretic.

OLDER ADULTS

We've described intergenerational or historical trauma and the transmission of such trauma to offspring and their children (see Chapter 2). Such transmission of traumatic stress can create symptoms of PTSD in the children of those who originally experienced such events. But what happens over the life course? Does the time of the trauma in an individual's life determine how the older adult is able to heal? What effects does early trauma have on an older adult's functioning later in life?

Oftentimes, we assume that with age comes resilience. Our mind-set is that older adults should have the wisdom from past life experiences to be able to process traumatic events in a different manner from those younger than themselves. The evidence suggests this superior ability to resolve trauma is dependent upon a number of factors.

A large national study that included data on 9,463 adults age 60 and older with lifetime PTSD found that these individuals had several physical illnesses compared with older adults who had experienced one or two traumatic events but did not meet criteria for PTSD (Pietrzak, Goldstein, Southwick, & Grant, 2012). These individuals were more likely to be diagnosed with hypertension, angina pectoris, tachycardia, other heart disease, stomach ulcer, gastritis, arthritis, and overall lower physical functioning than those not meeting PTSD criteria (odds ratios = 1.3–1.8; Pietrzak et al., 2012). Other researchers have revealed similar findings for PTSD that persists in later life. Byers, Covinsky, Neylan, and Yaffe (2014) analyzed data on 3,287 adults over 55 years of age. Controlling for several variables, including individual medical conditions and depression, those older adults with persistent PTSD were found to be three times more likely to have any disability when compared with individuals with no PTSD (Byers et al., 2014).

In another study, Petkus and colleagues (2018) found that in a sample of 76 older adults, a past history of childhood trauma was associated with worse performance on processing speed, attention, and executive functioning. Interestingly, cortisol levels were not associated with childhood trauma (in contrast to self-reports; Petkus, Lenze, Butters, Twamley, & Wetherell, 2018). Despite PTSD being common in the older adult population, acute traumatization symptom severity is generally lower in older than in younger groups. Further, early-life traumatic events appear to affect the older adult more so than late-life events; however, more research is needed to confirm this because the severity of the trauma is an important factor (Böttche, Kuwert, & Knaevelsrud, 2012).

Anderson, Fields, and Dobb (2011) assert that activities of daily living in long-term care facilities may be trauma triggers for older residents. They offer an example of an older adult who has experienced sexual abuse and is dependent on another for bathing. Another instance is when a Holocaust survivor needs assistance with undressing, providing a trigger to the past trauma of extreme fear and humiliation (Anderson et al., 2011). Using psychosocial assessments upon admission may be one way to reveal a history of past trauma; asking whether the individual has experienced trauma and describing various examples may be sufficient to assess this history (Anderson et al., 2011). What this means is that as nurses when we approach and assess older adults, their hidden past life events may play a role in their cognitive, physical, and behavioral functioning.

SECONDARY TRAUMATIC STRESS

In Chapter 2, we discussed secondary trauma and how secondary traumatic stress (STS) affects the caregiver, a burden that may lead to compassion fatigue. For example, a student nurse or nurse may experience secondary trauma of grieving families after the loss of a family member. Another example is the shock of a family receiving a terminal diagnosis for a young mother with breast cancer. Or comforting a coworker who has been hit by an incoherent patient and is awaiting X-ray results of a possible broken jaw. Each of these scenarios brings to the surface the secondary effects of trauma from witnessing trauma in others.

But how do you know if you're experiencing symptoms of STS? One tool, the Secondary Traumatic Stress Scale (STSS), developed by Brian Bride and colleagues (Bride et al., 2004), may be helpful (see Table 3.2). The tool was originally developed for social workers and others in the helping professions, including nurses, and contains 17 items that contribute to three subscales (intrusion, avoidance, and arousal). While modeling the scale after PTSD factors outlined in the DSM-4 (APA, 1994), the difference occurs in the wording so that the stressor is identified as "exposure to clients" (Bride et al., 2004, p. 29). Although there is no cutoff score when using the STSS, caregivers are asked to simply add their scores (1 = never to 5 = very often). In the case of nursing, the "client" may be a patient or a coworker.

TABLE 3.2   THE SECONDARY TRAUMATIC STRESS SCALE (STSS)

The following is a list of statements made by persons who have been impacted by their work with traumatized clients. Read each statement, and then indicate how frequently the statement was true for you in the past seven (7) days by circling the corresponding number next to the statement.

	NEVER	RARELY	OCCASIONALLY	OFTEN	VERY OFTEN
1. I felt emotionally numb.	1	2	3	4	5
2. My heart started pounding when I thought about my work with clients.	1	2	3	4	5
3. It seems as if I was reliving the trauma(s) experienced by my client(s).	1	2	3	4	5
4. I had trouble sleeping.	1	2	3	4	5
5. I felt discouraged about the future.	1	2	3	4	5
6. Reminders of my work with clients upset me.	1	2	3	4	5
7. I had little interest in being around others.	1	2	3	4	5
8. I felt jumpy.	1	2	3	4	5
9. I was less active than usual.	1	2	3	4	5
10. I thought about my work with clients when I didn't intend to.	1	2	3	4	5
11. I had trouble concentrating.	1	2	3	4	5

continues

73

TABLE 3.2 THE SECONDARY TRAUMATIC STRESS SCALE (STSS) (CONT.)

	NEVER	RARELY	OCCASIONALLY	OFTEN	VERY OFTEN
12. I avoided people, places, or things that reminded me of my work with clients.	1	2	3	4	5
13. I had disturbing dreams about my work with clients.	1	2	3	4	5
14. I wanted to avoid working with some clients.	1	2	3	4	5
15. I was easily annoyed.	1	2	3	4	5
16. I expected something bad to happen.	1	2	3	4	5
17. I noticed gaps in my memory about client sessions.	1	2	3	4	5

NOTE: "Client" is used to indicate persons with whom you have been engaged in a helping relationship. You may substitute another noun that better represents your work such as consumer, patient, recipient, and so forth.

Source: © 1999, Brian E. Bride; Reprinted with permission, Bride et al., 2004

From physiological changes (for example, "heart pounding" and "less active than usual") to cognitive awareness ("gaps in my memory") to intrusive thoughts ("I thought about my work"), we understand how the work of nursing may affect us as individuals in myriad ways. As we move forward on our journey and extend comfort to others, this simple assessment may be helpful to understand whether secondary traumatic stress is affecting us.

Additional scales have been used in nursing to measure compassion fatigue (a cumulative drain on our emotional resources). These include the

Compassion Fatigue Self Test for Helpers (Figley, 1995) and the Compassion Fatigue Scale–Revised, which is a modified version of the Compassion Fatigue Scale (Gentry, Baranowsky, & Dunning, 2002). Each scale has demonstrated acceptable validity and reliability in numerous studies.

ANOTHER SIDE TO THE COIN: US AS TRAUMA PERPETRATORS

In this section, we personalize the phenomenon of treatment trauma and look in the mirror to reflect whether we are culpable of traumatic stress in our patients. As a young nursing instructor, Karen was supervising the care of student nurses to a middle-aged woman who weighed 300 pounds. Her weight precluded her from standing independently, and she was from a disadvantaged socioeconomic group. Bologna and macaroni and cheese were commonly included in her diet. At the nurses' station, Karen overheard staff members snickering about the obese woman, making jokes of her condition. The woman had tearfully verbalized shame and humiliation at her appearance and her dependency on personal hygiene from others. The incident struck Karen as being mean-spirited, and also, the patient admitted to knowing she was being ridiculed, adding to the trauma the woman experienced while in the hospital.

At times, healthcare workers tend to objectify patients as a way of protecting themselves. When we do this, we become perpetrators of traumatic experiences, and a destructive cycle forms: patients are a diagnosis, a room number, described in ways that dehumanize them. As objects, we perform tasks to them, not with them. And we separate away from the humanistic experiences that enrich our souls and are the reasons we became nurses.

There are also times when we unintentionally show biases toward others, called *implicit biases*. To be a nurse, you have to know yourself (Carper, 1978; Chinn & Kramer, 2015), which can mean facing attitudes and beliefs that you value but that may show unconscious bias. It is important that you know yourself and your values; otherwise, you won't be aware of how you may affect others, whose beliefs differ.

TRAUMA-INFORMED REFLECTION

During your last clinical experience, was there an incident when a patient was objectified and defined by a diagnosis, a surgical procedure, a geographical location (room or unit), or another characteristic devoid of individualization? Did you stop to think about the label? Was the patient aware of the label? What if the patient had been aware? Do you think if we called patients in face-to-face interactions labels such as "the coronary angioplasty w/stent in room 301," we would alter our behaviors? Why would being present with the patient diminish such objectification?

Project Implicit (2011) is a nonprofit organization and collaboration of researchers who work together to understand implicit social cognition or "thoughts and feelings outside of conscious awareness and control" (para. 1). This project allows individuals to take task-based assessments that demonstrate preferences of various population traits or characteristics. For example, there are assessments on gender, sexuality, weight, race, ethnicity, age, and others. At the end of the assessment, you're offered your preference based on your performance (Project Implicit, 2011; see also https://www.projectimplicit.net/index.html). For example, Karen learned, based on this one-time performance assessment, that she has a moderate positive perception of young people versus older adults. This might be accurate because Karen primarily interacts with younger and middle-aged adults as an instructor and researcher.

The question is whether awareness will impact behaviors stemming from bias. We all arrive in the clinical world with our own personal inclinations formed by family, friends, and experiences. Our awareness of these inclinations becomes more pronounced when we process our reactions and take note of our actions that result from our patient interactions.

CONCLUSIONS

Just as trauma is an individual experience, so, too, is the way an individual processes trauma, contingent on internal and external factors. By accounting for ACEs (Felitti et al., 1998), we understand that childhood traumatic experiences represent a concerning presence in our world. The Event, Experience, and Effects (SAMHSA, 2014) reveal how trauma translates into daily life and should be situated within a developmental framework. Asking, "What has happened to you?" when assessing for traumatic events allows the patient to know there is opportunity to connect with others in a safe environment. Focusing on the nurse, we understand how secondary traumatic stress can negatively impact us both personally and professionally and can be assessed with a validated scale (Bride et al., 2004). Understanding that caregivers may be sources of trauma enables us to continually assess ourselves, and our conscious and implicit biases toward others.

HIGHLIGHTS OF CHAPTER CONTENT

- Adverse childhood experiences (ACEs) are dose-dependent events that present health risks into adulthood and have a startling presence in the US. Some situate ACEs as a public health crisis.

- Assessing individuals who have experienced trauma is based on how the Event, Experience, and Effects are assimilated and contingent on developmental factors.

- The nurse is a being who may be affected by the trauma of others (secondary traumatic stress), who may have experienced firsthand trauma, and is one who may inflict trauma onto others through actions and biases.

- Asking the trauma-informed question "What has happened to you?" allows for compassionate connections to form and opens a forum for healing to occur.

REFERENCES

American Psychiatric Association. (1994). *Diagnostic and statistical manual of mental disorders* (4th ed.). Washington, DC: Author.

American Psychiatric Association. (2013). *Diagnostic and statistical manual of mental disorders* (5th ed.). Arlington, VA: Author.

Anderson, K. A., Fields, N. L., & Dobb, L. A. (2011). Understanding the impact of early-life trauma in nursing home residents. *Journal of Gerontological Social Work, 54*(8), 755. doi: 10.1080/01634372.2011.596917

Bethell, C. D., Carle, A., Hudziak, J., Gombojav, N., Powers, K., Wade, R., & Braveman, P. (2017). Methods to assess adverse childhood experiences of children and families: Toward approaches to promote child well-being in policy and practice. *Academic Pediatrics, 17*(7), S51–S69.

Böttche, M., Kuwert, P., & Knaevelsrud, C. (2012). Posttraumatic stress disorder in older adults: An overview of characteristics and treatment approaches. *International Journal of Geriatric Psychiatry, 27*, 230–239. doi:10.1002/gps.2725

Bride, B. E., Robinson, M. M., & Yegidis, B. (2004). Development and validation of the Secondary Traumatic Stress Scale. *Research on Social Work Practice, 14*(1), 27–35. doi:10.1177/1049731503254106

Byers, A. L., Covinsky, K. E., Neylan, T. C., & Yaffe, K. (2014). Chronicity of posttraumatic stress disorder and risk of disability in older persons. *JAMA Psychiatry, 71*(5), 540–546. doi:10.1001/jamapsychiatry.2014.5

Carper, B. A. (1978). Fundamental patterns of knowing in nursing. *Advances in Nursing Science, 1*(1), 13–24. doi:10.1097/00012272-197810000-00004

Centers for Disease Control and Prevention. (n.d.). Adverse childhood experiences: Looking at how ACEs affect our lives and society. Retrieved from https://vetoviolence.cdc.gov/apps/phl/resource_center_infographic.html

Chinn, P., & Kramer, M. (2015). *Knowledge development in nursing: Theory and process* (9th ed.). St. Louis, MO: Mosby, Inc.

Felitti, V. J., & Anda, R. F. (2010). The relationship of adverse childhood experiences to adult medical disease, psychiatric disorders and sexual behavior: Implication for healthcare. In R. A. Lanius, E. Vermetten, & C. Pain (Eds.), *The impact of early life trauma on health and disease: The hidden epidemic* (pp. 77–87). New York, NY: Cambridge University.

Felitti, V. J., Anda, R. F., Nordenberg, D., Williamson, D. F., Spitz, A. M., Edwards, V., . . . Marks, J. S. (1998). Relationship of childhood abuse and household dysfunction to many of the leading causes of death in adults: The Adverse Childhood Experiences (ACE) study. *American Journal of Preventive Medicine, 14*(4), 245–258.

Figley, C. R. (1995). Compassion fatigue: Toward a new understanding of the costs of caring. In B. H. Stamm (Ed.), *Secondary traumatic stress: Self-care issues for clinicians, researchers, and educators* (pp. 3–28). Lutherville, MD: Sidran Press.

Gentry, J. E., Baranowsky, A. B., & Dunning, K. (2002). ARP: The Accelerated Recovery Program (ARP) for compassion fatigue. In C. R. Figley (Ed.), *Treating compassion fatigue* (pp. 123–137). New York, NY: Brunner-Rutledge.

National Child Traumatic Stress Network. (2010). Age-related reactions to a traumatic event. Retrieved from https://www.nctsn.org/sites/default/files/resources/age_related_reactions_to_traumatic_events.pdf

Petkus, A. J., Lenze, E. J., Butters, M. A., Twamley, E. W., & Wetherell, J. L. (2018). Childhood trauma is associated with poorer cognitive performance in older adults. *Journal of Clinical Psychiatry, 79*(1), 16m11021. doi:https://doi-org.ezproxy.lib.purdue. edu/10.4088/JCP.16m11021

Pietrzak, R. H., Goldstein, R. B., Southwick, S. M., & Grant, B. F. (2012). Physical health conditions associated with posttraumatic stress disorder in U.S. older adults: Results from Wave 2 of the National Epidemiologic Survey on Alcohol and Related Conditions. *Journal of the American Geriatrics Society, 60*, 296–303. doi:10.1111/ j.1532-5415.2011.03788.x

Project Implicit. (2011). About us. Retrieved from https://implicit.harvard.edu/implicit/ aboutus.html

Rahim, M. (2014). Developmental trauma disorder: An attachment-based perspective. *Clinical Child Psychology and Psychiatry, 19*(4), 548–560. doi:10.1177/1359104514534947

Sacks, V., & Murphey, D. (2018; updated February 20). *The prevalence of adverse childhood experiences, nationally, by state, and by race/ethnicity* [Research brief]. Retrieved from https://www.childtrends.org/wp-content/uploads/2018/02/ ACESBriefUpdatedFinal_ChildTrends_February2018.pdf

SAMSHA-HRSA Center for Integrated Health Solutions. (n.d.). Trauma. Retrieved from https://www.integration.samhsa.gov/clinical-practice/trauma-informed

Substance Abuse and Mental Health Services Administration. (2014). *SAMHSA's concept of trauma and guidance for a trauma-informed approach.* HHS Publication No. (SMA) 14-4884. Rockville, MD: Author.

Sun, T. (2018, January 30). Duck syndrome and a culture of misery. *The Stanford Daily.* Retrieved from https://www.stanforddaily.com/2018/01/31/duck-syndrome-and-a- culture-of-misery/

LEARNING OBJECTIVES

At the end of this chapter, you will be able to:

- Interpret Herman's (2015) three stages of individual recovery from trauma.

- Translate the stages of grief to the context of loss and grief surrounding trauma.

- Identify tangible and intangible losses that occur as a result of trauma and injury.

- Understand the different physical and psychological factors that contribute to an individual's resiliency and subsequent outcomes.

- Debate the quote "What doesn't kill me makes me stronger" (Nietzsche) within the context of trauma.

- Evaluate at least three ways individuals use to heal from trauma.

PURPOSE OF THE CHAPTER

We designed this book to increase self-awareness and awareness of trauma in others. We believe such self-awareness will impact the quality of life of and the quality of care rendered by students and new nurses. But this book is not designed as a textbook in the field of psychology to teach therapeutic techniques or interventions to recover from psychological trauma. In this chapter, we offer an overview and describe common approaches to healing from trauma so that you are aware of these

HEALING FROM PSYCHOLOGICAL TRAUMA: AN OVERVIEW

4

modalities. Although nurses pride themselves on the delivery of evidence-based care, mental health interventions are challenging to definitively list and evaluate. Indeed, the 2015 report issued by the Institute of Medicine on mental health interventions states:

> The levels and quality of evidential support vary widely across the myriad psychosocial interventions. This variation reflects a reality in the field. The evidence base for some psychosocial interventions is extensive, while that for others, even some that are commonly used, is more limited. (p. 26)

For the present, we focus on how you as an individual and as a nurse can apply trauma-informed interventions in your lives and practices. Still, we want to remain cognizant of the range of approaches to healing trauma, some of which are specific to special groups (for example, veterans and children in foster care), the levels of providers who deliver these approaches, and the setting of the interventions.

RECOVERING FROM THINGS AND PEOPLE THAT HURT US

How do people heal from individual trauma? How do they find the path to move forward in a new and sustained way and reappear from the darkness with knowledge and trust that there is still light in the world? Thousands of books and hundreds of articles have addressed this, and more will be written. We find a simple path may offer insight. And yet "path" may not be the best descriptor because as we recover, our journey takes us back and forth, forward and backward, with periods of feeling discouraged and then, renewed hope. Similar to the stages of grief articulated by Kübler-Ross and Kessler (2014), the process we, and those around us, move toward is iterative, sometimes frustratingly repetitive. Some of us get stuck and wait for an epiphany to move us. But looking behind us, we see progress that, at times, seems so very slow. We draw again from Herman (2015), in which she describes healing from trauma:

> Recovery unfolds in three stages. The central task of the first stage is the establishment of safety. The central task of the second stage is remembrance and mourning. The central task of the third stage is reconnection with ordinary life. (p. 155)

Reinforcing how brains react to stress and trauma, for many of us, the "off switch" comes in the form of feeling safe. What that means to each of us may vary. Physical safety is paramount and in some ways the most concrete to obtain. Psychological safety may be more complex to achieve and sustain. After trauma has occurred, we are on the lookout for it to reemerge. Trauma's unpredictability may have the individual in a state of hypervigilance, and we're motivated to be on the ready for its reemergence. Because of our efforts, we are exhausted.

Our quest in recovery is for feeling psychologically safe and sustaining this feeling. For many who have experienced trauma, this goal is only achieved when there is a consciousness that safety is the void they need to fill to continue the process of healing. Once the individual establishes that, in that moment, there is a place and space where injury is not a threat, the person is able to move to the second stage: remembrance and mourning.

Remembering pain can carry with it a renewal of trauma we desperately want to keep buried. It is a secret within ourselves, which for multiple and compelling reasons, we don't want shared. Injuries in childhood bring with them a special confusion, especially if the trauma was from those we should have been able to trust the most. But a part of us just as desperately wishes to expose, describe, feel, and, in the process, know that our humanness remains intact despite what has happened to us, what we have seen, and what we have endured. In our decades of experience, we have arrived at the conclusion that something is very healing in being able to share our experiences with others who are trustworthy. Once remembrance has occurred, our own private processing can take us only so far, and then, seeking out another can help us in new ways.

Selecting that person or persons to share with when trauma is present is a task that needs to be considered carefully. Often, the person with private trauma has a history of being cautious about whom to trust. Again, the feeling of safety is jeopardized when evaluating the connection with another. Perhaps the individual is a mental health professional, a trusted friend, or another family member. The right person who can listen to our story and understand what happened to us is therapeutic and renewing.

When there has been injury and trauma, there is a loss. Something was skewed in our lives, something taken. Sometimes there is no replacement for the loss, and with this realization, our grief can be overwhelming. Grief can bring many emotions, including sadness, anger, intermittent denial ("Did I remember that right?"), and ultimately, acceptance. Again, the work of Kübler-Ross and Kessler (2014), although evolved as a framework for the death of a loved one, may be applicable in the ways grief surrounding trauma is experienced: denial, anger, bargaining, depression, and acceptance. Within the context of trauma, the realization of the loss may trigger those stages (or some of those stages) to be experienced. In denial, we wonder whether the trauma was really traumatic. Or if a distant memory, we ask, "Did it really happen?" Anger may be directed at those who have harmed us or stolen something from us, such as childhood innocence. Or it may be channeled to others. However justified our anger may be, there is no justification to harming others. But keep in mind that anger alone is not a "bad" emotion. It can be healing and motivating. Bargaining is another way traumatic loss may be experienced. Perhaps it is a reconciliation or a pact: "If I do this, then X, Y, and Z will be better." It may justify substance use: "I need this to go on." It may also relate to how we see ourselves: "If I tell someone about my trauma, then I will be a better person." Depression is a human response to loss. As with other emotions, processing the depression moves us further along to acceptance. With trauma, we believe that acceptance is part of our healing. We accept a new way of living moving forward.

Regardless of the organizing framework, the losses must be mourned, be it the loss of:

- Untainted views of the world around you, the loss of innocence, trust, security

- Physical ability, resulting in an inability to perform or exist as a typical adult in society

- A home or space meant to be a special place to live in

- A competent, caring parent, such as in the cases of neglect or abuse

- Resources to ensure basic needs are met, such as housing, food, and clean clothing

- A passing or exit from your life of a loved family member or friend

- Living a life free of substance dependency

- Feeling that you are no longer the same as others/now "different" from others

- What was expected to come to you in life

TRAUMA-INFORMED REFLECTION

Think about a time when you lost an important possession or someone left your life—someone who was important to you. What were your emotions? Did your emotions map to the stages of grief (Kübler-Ross & Kessler, 2014)? How did you express or cope with denial or anger? Were these actions adaptive or maladaptive? Did you know at the time you were mourning a loss?

Emotions, for those who have endured trauma, are often feared. They may make the person uncomfortable, and by not feeling, the person avoids further pain and suffering. Or the person may not trust himself to regulate his emotions and decide to evade expressing emotions as an alternative. This sense of flawed safety denies the person the ability to move forward with his life. Unfortunately, this avoidance can also be in the form of self-medicating with substances, such as alcohol or other drugs. Numbing the pain through substance use may become substance dependency, abuse, and addiction. Recognizing health-defeating resilience is key to understanding reactions to trauma and supporting healing (Hunter & Chandler, 1999).

As with the grief we experience when death occurs, recovery from trauma allows us new opportunities to grow and encounter life with resiliency and compassion for others. But we can also become bitter and withdrawn if our mourning is unresolved. The third stage, reconnection with life, may be incredibly fulfilling. The person feels a sense of freedom from the trauma that has been carried psychologically for so long. He can now be the person of his own choosing, unencumbered by the darkness that was hidden. Although the individual may now face life with insight and gentleness toward himself and others, he is changed by his past. And something positive emerges from trauma: strength and awareness.

Folks who have come out from the other side of a traumatic experience with renewed self-worth and compassion receive the gift of survivorship and more. It's the "more" that is important: the ability to have fully experienced the human condition and to understand others in a way that often instills a desire to treat others with kindness and true empathy.

So returning to our "ordinary life" (Herman, 2015, p. 155) may mean creating a new ordinary life, which may be a good thing because our past life may not be psychologically compatible any longer. There is emotional work to be done in letting go of what has protected us in the past and allowed us to function in daily life. We now know the origins of our behaviors, actions, and perceptions born from trauma and injurious experiences. We are on the journey to making sense of our lives; this journey changes us and how we see the world and our role in it. Our goals may change. People in our lives may be viewed differently. The issue of forgiveness of others' transgressions against us, those who have been the source of trauma, is complex and individualized.

Commonly, we connect a spiritual dimension to forgiveness of others. Often, we need to first forgive ourselves and place past thoughts and behaviors within a context of traumatic experiences. Seeing the links between present and past behaviors through this trauma lens can support our journey to forgiveness. Some mental health professionals believe that in certain circumstances, forgiveness may not be possible. We believe it is a decision that is made with time and by the individual based on specific circumstances of past events.

One of the challenges during our reentry into an ordinary life is to avoid becoming too egocentric or self-involved, but rather to feel a sense of worth that is new and held with conviction. We work hard to begin to trust ourselves, become centered, with an innate clarity of who we are. There can be a temptation to believe our enduring and surviving trauma has made us superior to others. We may be lured into thinking that we are somehow "tougher," "stronger," or have evolved into a state others may not be able to accomplish.

With time, there is a contentment, a psychological settling in, and a new beginning to our ordinary lives. We have the opportunity to engage with others, our interactions colored by humility, insight, and compassion. We know now, after all, that each of us has a story, a narrative, which so often describes something in our past that is called "trauma." We are not alone in this.

TRAUMA-INFORMED REFLECTION

Think of a time when someone in your life, or you, reached out to another person to share an emotional experience. Perhaps it was a particularly happy day or memory. Or it may have been a difficult personal or professional day. How did sharing with someone make you feel? How important was the reaction of the other person? What did you seek from the person you were sharing with? How do patients share with nurses who care for them? What are they seeking?

RESILIENCY AND PSYCHOLOGICAL GROWTH

Resiliency is a big part of understanding how to recover and heal from trauma. Consider two nursing students who are studying for their senior year final examinations in public health nursing. This is their final semester, and both need at least a B on the exam to pass the course.

One student, Lindsey, has been faced with myriad challenges throughout the year. Her mother was diagnosed with stage II ovarian cancer and received several rounds of chemotherapy. The toxicities of the chemotherapy agents left her mother in a cognitive fog and dramatically changed the once close relationship Lindsey had enjoyed with her. Her father, dependent upon his wife for keeping the household running, had shut down, spending hours in the basement watching TV and drinking beer after coming home from work. Lindsey recently broke up with her boyfriend of six months, who "was feeling a lot of negative energy from her." Through attempts to "medicate" her anxiety through alcohol, she performed poorly on the first three exams and now was feeling the pressure of this last exam that determined whether she would graduate.

The second student, Maggie, also had faced adversity this past year. Last summer, she'd witnessed several patients pass away while working as a nursing assistant in a rural, acute care hospital; several of these individuals she'd known her whole life. Intrusive thoughts often played out in her mind—scenes of patients dying with families weeping around the bedside and insufficient staff members to meet patient needs. The realities of nursing had become too apparent, overwhelming her emotions at times. In her personal life, her brother had become involved in substance use, buying opioids from dealers, caused from a painful and lingering injury he'd sustained while playing football in high school. Now homeless, he would randomly call to ask for money and berate her when she refused or explained she didn't have any to give him. She didn't see her father very often, as her parents divorced four years ago, but Maggie remembers his "go for it!" attitude. Her mother wasn't a big part of her life and worked most of the time to meet the family's financial responsibilities. To enhance Maggie's test performance, her 16-year-old sister, whom Maggie was close to, had recently offered her some amphetamines, which had been prescribed for attention deficit problems. Her peers at school had seen the changes in Maggie, but she'd declined their offers to "talk." Feeling distracted and anxious, even paralyzed with fear, Maggie slept or played video games to cope. She attended class but was disengaged. On a partial scholarship, Maggie would lose funding if she failed the class and had to postpone graduation. Maggie was all too aware of what the next three weeks meant to her career and life.

Both had three weeks left to study. Both had experienced traumatic events or witnessed traumatic events endured by others.

A TALE OF TWO STUDENTS AND RESILIENCY

Here, we track those three weeks for each of the students leading up to the final exam and examine the role of resiliency.

Lindsey's anxiety heightened. Despite wanting to avoid alcohol, she continued to drink alone, hiding it from others. She isolated herself from friends and family, and from peers and faculty at school. Days and nights were turned around, and she could barely make it to class. Her identity and self-esteem had been contingent on having a boyfriend, and she'd overlooked many of his faults to be in the relationship. Now, looking back, she kept thinking how even a "loser" like him didn't want her. She ruminated on how she'd never been a strong student, except in the peds class, where she had wanted to obtain a position. But graduating looked like an impossible goal she probably wasn't capable of achieving. Her only support, her mom, was gone, at least for now, and she wondered if she were really more like her father. Lindsey failed the exam and did not graduate. When the nursing student advisor insisted on meeting with her to talk about next steps, Lindsey didn't show up.

Maggie felt as if someone had finally woken her up from a deep sleep. Of course, nursing was what she wanted! She committed to preparing for the test over the next three weeks to ensure she'd pass. She was convinced she could and would. Next, she went to her sister, gently thanking her for her willingness to help her get through the long hours of studying that were ahead. But Maggie also emphasized to her sister that she should only take the medication herself and as it was prescribed. An awareness also began to grow in her that her brother's problems were affecting her. She assessed herself and knew she had signs of depression. So, she reached out to her peers and asked to study with them. Maggie emailed her course instructor for guidance on studying for the final and shared this information with her study group. One of her friends told her about the campus counseling center, where she was assessed and awaiting her first appointment. At the session a few days later, she described how terribly guilty she felt toward not helping her brother. The theme of helplessness at witnessing patients' deaths and her brother's addiction became clear. She'd even adopted that same helpless behavior in school, which now threatened her future. This insight supported her efforts to prepare for the final, which she was able to pass. Maggie graduated on time and accepted a position as a staff nurse on an inpatient psychiatric unit.

UNDERSTANDING RESILIENCY THROUGH CONCEPT ANALYSES

Now, we review the literature and map these two cases to the characteristics of resiliency. We begin with one of the best approaches to describing an abstract concept: a concept analysis.

Garcia-Dia, DiNapoli, Garcia-Ona, Jakubowski, and O'Flaherty (2013) examined the concept of resilience and listed its attributes as rebounding, social support, and self-efficacy. Rebounding was described as the ability to bounce back, metaphorically, for the person not to be broken by the trauma or event. Determination or the intention of overcoming was also important in having resilience. Having social support is a common factor in much of the psychological literature and mitigates several negative outcomes, including depression. The belief that one can overcome trauma through self-efficacy was also a recurrent pattern uncovered in the analysis (Garcia-Dia et al., 2013). A definition was proposed for resilience:

> one's ability to bounce back or recover from adversity.
> It is a dynamic process that can be influenced by the environment, external factors, and/or the individual and the outcome.
> (p. 267)

In this definition, the interplay between the individual and environment is noted. In a more recent concept analysis of resilience, Niitsu and colleagues (2017) integrate genetics into the analysis. The addition of *heredity* connects an individual's resilience to various genes carried by reproduction. The authors link specific genes to regulation of brain circuitry and the hypothalamic-pituitary-adrenal axis function, which they hypothesize may affect an individual's resilience (Niitsu et al., 2017). The interplay between genes and environment is also emphasized. The attributes or characteristics revealed were ego-resiliency, emotion regulation, social support, and heredity (Niitsu et al., 2017, p. 898). The proposed definition of resilience is:

> a dynamic process of positive adaptation following exposure to PTEs, facilitated by ego-resiliency, emotion regulation, social support, and heredity, and evidenced by none to mild psychopathological symptoms and positive adaptation through development of a SOC. (Niitsu et al., 2017, p. 902)

Note: PTE = potentially traumatic event; SOC = sense of coherence.

In an autobiographical analysis, Dekel (2017) describes her "truisms" related to resilience on three levels: the individual, the couple, and the community:

- On an individual level, "maintaining self-differentiation and retaining emotional boundaries" (p. 10) are necessary to be resilient. Being able to self-differentiate contributes to less reactivity, less stress, and less avoidant behaviors.

- At the couple level (spouse or caregiver), being able to make sense of and find meaning in the experience contributes to resiliency and even posttraumatic growth.

- At the community level, feeling that an individual belongs to a group that will support his needs and one that the individual feels an emotional attachment toward supports the ability to cope with stress and greater resiliency.

Extrapolating from Dekel's conclusions, we can see that nurses as a group could strengthen resiliency through a sense of community belonging. In Chapter 2, we discussed workplace violence, incivility, and oppression. Each of these may be mitigated through efforts to ensure the individual has needs met, support, and a feeling that peers "have my back" in stressful times.

Resilience may be viewed as a trait, a process, a defense mechanism, or an outcome, depending upon the context, the resources available, and the individual. Resilience is also related to compassion fatigue and burnout, with an inverse relationship (the higher the resilience, the lower the compassion fatigue and burnout; Burnett, 2017). The question remains: How does the presence of resilience protect us, defend us, and accomplish these optimal outcomes?

Think back to Lindsey and Maggie. Lindsey wasn't able to pass the test, but Maggie was. While there were many issues that both young adults faced, Maggie demonstrated resilience by being able to rebound from the initial trauma and secondary trauma she'd experienced (resilience as a trait). She was convinced she could reach her goal and was able to regulate her emotions when she spoke to her sister. She mobilized her resources by studying with her friends and utilizing the campus counseling services (resilience as a process). The insights gained allowed her to look at her life in a new and growth-enhancing way (resilience as an outcome). Perhaps her father's "go for it!" way of thinking/personality had been reproductively and genetically passed on to Maggie.

In contrast, Lindsey's self-efficacy, ego-resiliency, and ability to rebound were lacking. Added to this, she'd lost several important sources of social and emotional support. First, she'd lost her close relationship to her mother, and her father's behaviors indicated disengagement and potential substance abuse, maladaptive coping with potential genetic components. Her boyfriend, who may not have ultimately been an authentic source of support, had boosted her self-esteem, albeit temporarily. However, the loss of his presence contributed to her lack of resilience. Both cases reflect viewing resilience as a trait (something we have), a process (something we do), and an outcome (some result).

> ## TRAUMA-INFORMED REFLECTION
>
> How resilient are you? Think of a time, event, or experience that was difficult for you. Were you able to rebound from it? Did the attributes described in the two concept analyses of resilience influence how well you recovered from the occurrence (Garcia-Dia et al. [2013]: rebounding, social support, and self-efficacy; Niitsu et al. [2017]: ego-resiliency, emotion regulation, social support, and heredity)?

POSTTRAUMATIC GROWTH

Posttraumatic growth, originally developed through the work of Tedeschi and Calhoun, has also been empirically identified as a potential outcome from a traumatic experience (Turner, Hutchinson, & Wilson, 2018). In the posttraumatic growth model, the aftermath of trauma and valuing what has been experienced and how coping has been used to survive is key; however, the trauma may remain distressing (Tedeschi & Calhoun, 2004). This sentiment is captured in Friedrich Nietzsche's (1844–1900) famous quote: "What doesn't kill me makes me stronger." Nietzsche was a German philosopher and scholar who has been significantly influential in Western philosophy and history. In this quote, Nietzsche seems to be saying that there are two paths when one encounters the traumas of life: death or an existence of higher strength. Colman (2015) defines posttraumatic growth as:

> Improvement in psychological functioning following a traumatic experience, especially in the areas of self-evaluation (increased self-confidence and acceptance of personal limitations), personal relationships (increased compassion, appreciation of intimacy, and appreciation of friendships), and personal philosophy (replacement of materialistic outlook with deeper understanding of what matters in life). (n.p.)

Nested within positive psychology, posttraumatic growth extends us an opportunity to come through difficult times with more than what we had before—be it awareness of self or of our relationships with others—and a transformed personal philosophy. In a study conducted by Li, Cao, Cao, and Liu (2015), nursing students' posttraumatic growth was associated with emotional intelligence and psychological resilience. Interestingly, curvilinear models (versus linear relationships) suggest that moderate emotional intelligence and moderate psychological resilience are associated with the most growth (Li et al., 2015). These results suggest that too much (high) or too little (low) emotional intelligence or resilience are not as strongly associated with posttraumatic growth.

How do we measure or know whether growth has occurred? Personal reflection, a feeling of being centered and a newfound contentment with life, and new dynamics in interpersonal communications may all provide internal evidence of growth. In addition, one tool that has been developed within the framework of positive psychology is the Posttraumatic Growth Inventory (PTGI), originally developed by Tedeschi and Calhoun (1995, 1996). This is a 21-item inventory designed to measure changes after a traumatic event in the following areas: new possibilities, relating to others, personal strength, appreciation of life, and spiritual change (Tedeschi & Calhoun, 1995, 1996). A new version of this tool expands spiritual change to encompass a "spiritual-existential change" that represents broader cultural experiences. This new tool, the Posttraumatic Growth Inventory-X, has 25 items (4 new items based on the spiritual-existential expanded dimension) and shows validity in a wider international context (Tedeschi, Cann, Taku, Senol-Durak, & Calhoun, 2017).

HEALED FROM TRAUMA: THE LIVED EXPERIENCE

One of the phrases we see used frequently is "the lived experience." It is another way of describing a personal experience that has influenced you in different ways. The phrase also imparts legitimacy to the individual-biographical; our personal understanding because of what we've lived has validity and importance. As an individual first and a nurse second, you will need to heal from the raw wounds left by trauma and understand how they affect you, and therefore, how they influence the comfort you offer to others. There are descriptions of coming out of trauma, as if we walk through a gate or portal and emerge from the other side a different being.

That's kind of the goal, as long as the person who has walked through that gate is able to feel more compassion, more depth, and an ability to give yet ensure that her emotional tank is filled as well. It is the enlightenment of a different way of living: knowing that bad things cannot be avoided, nor the unexpectedness of them. But it is also knowing that, in the end, things will be OK. This new state may not be what we initially wanted or even hoped for, but OK nonetheless. It is a peaceful way to think and one that allows fear to be experienced in measured doses as compared to living in a constant state of apprehension and dread.

INDIVIDUAL STRATEGIES

We frame the following descriptions of strategies, not as medical prescriptions or substitutes for therapy or professional provider management. Further, this section is not meant to be an exhaustive discussion about the various paths toward healing from trauma. Therefore, we outline and offer a general overview of select treatment modalities related to trauma recovery that we believe are most helpful at this stage in your career and for which your skill set enables you to convey to others. Several of these approaches serve to support recovery from additional mental health diagnoses and disorders, such as depression and anxiety.

RELATIONSHIPS/SOCIAL SUPPORT

The heading of this section might be a bit confusing. Is having a relationship a strategy to overcoming trauma? Not exactly. However, understanding the critical importance of positive relationships in our lives is significant because social support is able to mitigate the lasting effects of adverse life events. Attachment to others—being reciprocated in a healthy relationship—is integral to recovery. Further, it is one of the steps in healing by reconnecting with life.

Our earliest form of social support and our most influential relationship begins with our parents. Buffers to reduce traumatic effects may include parental responsiveness to children at high risk, even at the biomarker level. Asok, Bernard, Roth, Rosen, and Dozier (2013) found that higher parental response predicted increased telomere length in high-risk young children. The authors concluded that this "high-quality" parental relationship was significant in "modifying the biological impact of early-life stress" (Asok et al., 2013, p. 581). But how do relationships affect stress symptoms after maltreatment? What is it about the relationships with supportive caregivers that positively impacts children?

Another study may point in the right direction. Münzer, Ganser, and Goldbeck (2017) examined perceived social support, "maltreatment-related negative cognitions related to the 'worse' experience of maltreatment," and posttraumatic stress symptoms (PTSS; p. 183). These researchers found that the influence of cognitive coping through social interactions within relationships decreased PTSS. The children and adolescents had fewer negative beliefs about themselves and the world, shaped by participation in supportive relationships (Münzer et al., 2017). Using data from the National Survey of Child and Adolescent Well-Being, Yoon (2018) adds to these findings in a study of 449 children with a history of maltreatment. The author conducted a longitudinal study, tracking children over an eight-year period. Conclusions forwarded by the researcher are that children are fairly resilient. To add to positive outcomes, prosocial skill development (for example, self-control, responsibility) and caregiver well-being should be emphasized (Yoon, 2018). Thus, our ability to perceive ourselves and the world around us is shaped in a potentially healing way for children and adolescents who have been maltreated when they interact with supportive people. To optimize relationships, caregivers' well-being needs to be recognized and supported.

For adults, the type of social support is of note. Informal social support has been found to be more effective than formal social support for 150 adults who survived terror attacks in Israel. Informal support contributed to psychological improvement; however, formal support didn't produce these effects (Weinberg, 2017). These findings lead us to consider the type and quality of social support. Is the support from those who have experienced similar trauma and can identify with the trauma? Do women and men who have experienced trauma also experience social support differently? And even for perceived social support, does the source of informal social support matter (for example, family versus friends; see Evans, Steel, & DiLillo, 2013)?

As the Event, Experience, and Effects (Substance Abuse and Mental Health Services Administration [SAMHSA], 2014) vary with individuals, so, too will our needs as we seek ways and persons to help us heal. There is no "prescription" for ordering social support. As we begin to trust and seek someone safe to trust in, we need to avoid retraumatization and invest in those who will honor our needs.

JOURNALING/NARRATION

There is often something healing about putting thoughts to paper (even electronic "paper"). Perhaps it is our way of understanding our past through reflection and insight into the contexts of the past. One strategy is narrative discourse, chronicling our trauma so that a new coherence is made and moving forward is possible. Many memoirs found in the literature bear the mark of trauma narrations. They move us to understand the events, the injuries, and the recovery.

Several trauma-informed approaches use daily diaries, journaling, and narrative therapy as therapeutic ways to enter into and resolve traumatic events. Some argue that mastery, unity, and coherence are impossible and that such narratives can only exist in response to others within a context of power (Borg, 2018). Others argue that by telling our stories, we regain ownership over what was lost in trauma. If you decide that journaling or creating a trauma narration might be helpful to you, consider the following:

- Identify the emotions in your writing. Does the writing elicit feelings that are uncomfortable? How does confronting the trauma help you? What may precipitate the emotions?

- Think about memories that your writing brings. Where does the "story" begin and end? A crucial exercise is to tell your story and recall thoughts, feelings, and sensations.

- Consider drawing a picture or other representation of the trauma. What have you emphasized in the representation? Does this emphasis surprise you? How do you interpret the objects and their relationship to other objects in the drawing?

- Decide whether you'll share this information, and if so, with whom. This is a decision that is highly individualized based on several factors, including the degree of trust, the type of relationship, and the timing of the disclosure.

TRAUMA-INFORMED REFLECTION

Did you have a creative outlet for expressing yourself when you were younger (for example, writing, painting pottery, enjoying nature, collecting objects, or earning badges in youth clubs)? What did these activities do for your younger self? Did you feel rejuvenated when you were finished? If you stopped, do you miss it? Now, as an adult, how do you restore your energy when it is depleted?

MINDFULNESS

With its origins in Buddhist philosophy, mindfulness has become part of complementary medicine for addressing stress, crisis, and myriad psychological issues. One of the most prolific writers on the subject of mindfulness, Jon Kabat-Zinn (2015), defines mindfulness as:

> Mindfulness can be thought of as moment-to-moment, non-judgmental awareness, cultivated by paying attention in a specific way, that is, in the present moment, and as non-reactively, as non-judgmentally, and as openheartedly as possible. (p. 1481)

Mindfulness is also part of how we view pain and suffering. Shinzen Young (1994) forwarded a well-known equation to help us capture the Buddhist philosophy of these phenomena: "Suffering equals pain multiplied by resistance" or "$S = P \times R$" (pp. 58–59). This psychological formula is interpreted to mean that pain is universal and unavoidable. It is to be expected in life. Suffering, however, is considered optional, depending upon the resistance to pain we experience. Separating the two is often not apparent unless we begin to think about the phenomenon as distinct, with pain being experienced first and then resistance (which is optional) to that pain, and ultimately suffering. Being mindful, being insightful, and ultimately being free creates less (or no) suffering through less (or no) resistance. Young (1994) asserts:

> A spiritual insight is like a many-faceted jewel. One facet is called freedom from suffering. We can't avoid pain, but we certainly can avoid pain as a problem. (p. 59)

In this discussion, pleasure is also described as being "grasped" (Young, 1994, p. 59) by craving after the initial pleasure is experienced. Once the individual lets go of the craving, satisfaction from pleasure is realized (Young, 1994). When trauma affects us, we risk craving pleasure when our pain creates overwhelming suffering. Being mindful of these forces within us may support new insight that results in new behaviors.

MINDFULNESS MEDITATION AND QUIET SPACES

Various forms of meditation and multiple phone applications can help us incorporate meditation into our daily routines. Specific to nurses, in a pilot study with 15 nurses, Hevezi (2016) found that meditation five times per week over a six-month period resulted in higher compassion satisfaction and a decrease in burnout and secondary trauma. These results are supported in an integrative review of 16 articles that describe the effects of mindful meditation on nurses and nursing students (van der Rieta, Levett-Jones, & Aquino-Russell, 2018). In summary, the authors report that mindful meditation was positively impactful on stress, anxiety, depression, burnout, sense of well-being, and empathy (van der Rieta et al., 2018). The results are to be consumed, however, knowing that the reviewed studies are characterized by small sample sizes in single study sites.

A specific type of meditation that includes repetition of short phrases, called *mantram repetition,* involves softly repeating words while meditating. From the ancient language Sanskrit, one accepted translation of mantram is "instrument of thought." Several theories have been suggested on how mantram meditation works: distraction from troubling or negative stimuli and therefore, the creation of a new spiritual pathway. In this way, new energy is opened to us.

Bormann, Hurst, and Kelly (2013); Bormann, Oman, Walter, and Johnson (2014); and Bormann, Thorp, Wetherell, Golshan, and Lang (2013) have found that mantram meditation decreases symptoms of PTSD (such as nightmares and flashbacks), reduces depression, and increases feelings of well-being in veterans. Selecting a phrase is central to this meditation. Bormann (2014) recommends carefully selecting an existing phrase instead of inventing one and trying it for several weeks to see whether it is a good fit for meditation. If it isn't, a new mantram can be chosen. Mantrams are to be used over the lifetime; Bormann et al. (2014) suggest that the longer one is used, the more powerful it becomes.

Increasingly, nursing units have created "quiet room" spaces where nurses can refocus and process emotions before returning to the bedside. These might also be spaces for quick meditation exercises to occur.

DAILY STRUCTURE AND CIRCADIAN RHYTHM

From children to adults, evidence across the life span supports that sleep may be disrupted because of traumatic experiences. However, this isn't a constant finding; some individuals have difficulty with sleep, and others don't. Researchers are now beginning to understand why. Recall that one of the clusters of symptoms related to PTSD is hyperarousal (American Psychiatric Association, 2013). These symptoms include increased arousal, difficulty falling or staying asleep, increased irritability, outbursts of anger, difficulty concentrating, easily startled, and being hypervigilant.

A group of researchers believe that the inconsistency of findings related to sleep and PTSD can be found by looking at hyperarousal. In a preliminary study, van Wyk, Thomas, Solms, and Lipinska (2016) studied 57 female volunteers who were divided into four groups: PTSD with hyperarousal, PTSD without hyperarousal, depressive symptoms, and healthy control. Findings were as the group had hypothesized: Group 1, those with PTSD and hyperarousal, had the most disrupted sleep. More research is needed to investigate whether these specific symptoms of PTSD are related to poor sleep and, if so, to test interventions focused on these symptoms.

For many young adults, computer and phone screen time is part of daily life. More so, it is part of you—with many individuals literally and constantly plugged into the technology being used. It may be difficult to know when to flip the off switch. Overuse may have negative effects on weight, physical activity, and sleep. Our internal clock, our circadian rhythm, is the largest regulatory system in our body, keyed by light-dark and feeding-fasting cycles (Panda, 2016, p. 1008). Its disruption has significant implications for several adverse health outcomes related to metabolism: obesity, glucose intolerance/insulin resistance, cardiovascular diseases, chronic inflammation, liver diseases, increased cancer risk, and sleep disorders (Panda, 2016). Therefore, as we consider healing from trauma, our knowledge of the restorative powers of sleep and the timing of consumption of food are significant factors to consider.

AVOIDING HARMFUL SELF-MEDICATING

We live in a society when, at the end of a provider visit, we have come to expect a prescription for medication or treatment. The "wait and see" approach is usually not what many of us are satisfied with. Nor is it common to have individuals accept lifestyle changes as the "script" given to them. In some cases, the individual who has experienced trauma may avoid providers, hiding a secret that has been internalized.

In his practice, John will see young adults who attempt to self-medicate with illegal substances, including underage drinking, in an attempt to deaden the pain they are experiencing or running from. At times, it becomes a vicious cycle of using drugs to decrease depressive symptoms and enhance performance and then using other substances to relax and sleep. Students will visit John, pleading for an excuse to withdraw from class due to poor performance. What the students really need is to recognize the impact of the substance use on their lives. There is much to lose in these cases: health (vital signs are often abnormal, including elevated blood pressure); placement in school or employment; relationships; and time. Coming to terms with past trauma may be compounded when substance use dependence is a dual diagnosis.

HUMAN-ANIMAL BONDS AND INTERACTIONS

Many of you probably grew up with pets in your household. Evidence supports the healing powers of animals, from reducing stress to calming us. Animals helping us recover from trauma falls into the complementary medicine category. Two further delineations may be made (Pichot, 2013):

- Animal-assisted activities, commonly referred to as service dogs, are covered under the Americans with Disabilities Act and help humans perform tasks they cannot perform due to a disability. These animals are highly trained to perform functions to close the gap of the disability.

- Animal-assisted therapy (AAT) is described as use of animals in structured therapy. Individuals with developmental disorders, mental illnesses, and older adults with dementia have been shown to benefit from AAT (see Wynn, 2015, for further description).

Florence Nightingale is credited for being "the first known clinician to study animals in healthcare" (Pichot, 2013). Nightingale (2009) wrote:

2. A small pet animal is often an excellent companion for the sick, for long chronic cases especially. A pet bird in a cage is sometimes the only pleasure of an invalid confined for years to the same room. If he can feed and clean the animal himself, he ought always to be encouraged to do so. (Endnotes, p. 153)

We still have much to learn about the human-animal connection and the healing from trauma that may be gained. In the "Rebounding From Trauma" sidebar, we recount one of our pets: our dog, Tony. He is special because he came to us having experienced the trauma of being "dumped" by his first owner and being mistaken as aggressive.

OUR DOG, TONY: REBOUNDING FROM TRAUMA

We love dogs and have included dogs as part of our family since we have been a couple. There is something special about them and their ability to take in our stress and offer us a calming presence. One dog in particular has been an important member of our household for 11 years. His name is Tony, and this is his story.

At the time, we were living in a home with 10 acres of land, located about 20 minutes outside of a large city. For several days, we happened to see a large black and brown dog, clearly a Rottweiler mix, who must have been drawn to our home because of our other three dogs. He frightened us because of his size and his overall appearance, including a metal chain/choker collar. The farmer next door had been trying to catch him for weeks, annoyed with him and the disruption the dog was causing on his property. Finally, the farmer had installed a trap to capture the animal and planned to have animal control take him to be euthanized.

We were sitting in our living room when our dogs began to bark and become agitated. We looked out to see the dog on our front porch. Despite Karen's protests, John went outside and began soothing the dog, who had hidden himself behind our wicker furniture. He allowed John to pet him and seemed relieved to be in the presence of humans. We separated the dogs to allow the Rottweiler to relax and eat.

Soon, the family decided, what was one more dog? All four of them had become a pack.

Our son, Peter, named him "Tony," whose free spirits were matched. Tony was sick from eating parasitic-infected animal remains to survive. His throat had been damaged from the collar, and he was skittish at first. The vet examined him, prescribed a variety of anti-parasitic medications and antibiotics, and determined him to be about 9 months old. Tony soon looked at us with warm, brown eyes, but Karen couldn't help thinking that he was one of the ugliest dogs she'd ever seen. His snout was elongated, and he didn't have the body of the breed; her expectations were to see a Rottweiler, not a mixed breed.

Yet, within a few weeks, what he looked like didn't matter. Slowly, we became acquainted with each other. What surfaced was his intelligence and speed. He could outrun our invisible fence and quickly learned to outsmart the shock his collar tried to give to him for crossing the property boundaries. He became alpha with our other dogs and enjoyed being a benevolent leader.

Now, almost 11 years later, Tony has outlived several of our other dogs and remains a faithful, loving, protective, and grateful dog. He's put on a few pounds and can't run as fast as before, but he gives us more than we've ever given him: a caring presence; a being to hug, talk to, jump with; an animal that reciprocates love with a steady gaze, a tail wag, and a soft lick on the hand.

FINDING PURPOSE AND MEANING IN LIFE

Each of us has a different perception of a spiritual being, and some of us reject such a notion or are unsure. We may rest our beliefs on the universe and the patterns we suspect surround us. Whatever it is that provides us with reflection of a larger existence, many individuals who have experienced trauma find comfort in believing in a higher purpose and/or being. If we recall the work of Tedeschi and Calhoun (1995, 1996, 2004) in developing the posttraumatic growth model, you understand there is a new appreciation and value placed on the experience of trauma and the coping skills that emerged. One domain identified in posttraumatic growth is spiritual development (Tedeschi & Calhoun, 1996). The question remains as to the relationship between posttraumatic growth and psycho-spiritual transformation (Bray, 2010). The individual may need to make sense of trauma and position the event(s) in a broader spiritual context so that such posttraumatic growth may occur. For some of us, it is an existential question, helping us to make sense of what has happened and why we are here (Bray, 2010).

ADDITIONAL THOUGHTS ABOUT INDIVIDUAL STRATEGIES

In the previous sections, we describe some, but certainly not all, of the ways a person can begin to heal from trauma. Some of the strategies we've presented are approaches, some are tools, and some require changing an aspect of our environment. Please be aware that many more ways can be used to recover from trauma. Because this book is intended for individuals new to nursing, we believe these strategies represent a solid beginning to many future conversations you will have in your personal and professional journeys.

We also want to emphasize an important first step: recognizing that something has happened that you have evaluated as traumatic. Such recognition may not be readily apparent to the individual. It may be as Herman (2015) describes: a secret, kept both from ourselves and others. To heal from trauma, the person needs to acknowledge that something isn't right—about how she values herself, how she conducts herself, and how she views the world. To say this takes courage would be an understatement. To say embarking on a journey of recovery is hard work would minimize just how difficult it can be. But here's one thing we are certain of: To break the cycle that is perpetuated by trauma, these efforts are critical and can positively impact us as individuals and also those in our lives.

A WORD ABOUT APPS

Most of you reading this book are *digital natives,* meaning you grew up with technology as part of your space (Prensky, 2001). For you, using technology isn't necessarily novel or out of the ordinary. In contrast, technology immigrants didn't grow up and develop alongside of technology (Prensky, 2001). Many of the students we interact with will state that there is a marked difference in the use and ease with which technology is used and taken up between the two groups. We would also venture to state that technology immigrants are more skeptical of the use of technology and, at times, more readily see its limitations. Accessible information, needed education for the masses (for example, MOOCS—massive open online courses), and even enhancements to our mental health are some of the advances that technology offers. Millions of applications, or apps, are available to download. From games to fitness tracking to mental health support, apps are both a big business and an integration into daily life. But how do you know whether the app you're wanting to use has real value?

Some apps are specific to mental health. These application categories include:

- Meditation
- Mood disorders
- Obsessive compulsive disorder
- Stress and anxiety
- PTSD
- Schizophrenia
- Fears and phobias
- Eating disorders

In this context, it is important for you, as a consumer of a mental health app, to be a smart shopper. Has the application been tested to be effective? How transparent is it? What happens to the data/information you supply for tracking progress? One tool that may be beneficial is PsyberGuide (2018; https://psyberguide.org), a not-for-profit entity that evaluates various applications with different criteria (credibility, user experience, and transparency). Be vigilant when you use app technology in the same way you would with other technology—quality and cost vary, as does the amount of engagement with the user.

HEALING ADULTS, YOUTH, AND CHILDREN WHO HAVE BEEN AFFECTED BY TRAUMA

Although it is beyond the scope of this book to discuss the formal treatment modalities that are endorsed as evidence-based in helping those to heal from trauma, we acknowledge these as an imprecise yet important science. In addition to symptom management, most treatment modalities focus on core areas related to trauma and toxic stress in children, youth, and adults: attachment, emotional regulation, feeling competent, and forming healthy connections. The range of approaches is wide, from therapeutic play with children to grief counseling to eye movement desensitization and reprocessing (Shapiro, 1995/2001) to cognitive behavioral therapy (Beck, 2011).

As nurses, it is important you are aware of these therapeutic modalities; however, they are implemented by advanced practice nurses, social workers, psychologists, psychiatrists, and other mental health professionals. SAMHSA provides clinicians with a registry of evidence-based models for both adults and children: the Evidence-Based Practices Resource Center (SAMHSA, 2018). This portal allows you to search for best practice interventions by group and by audience. The guiding principle is once again based upon the individual; the type, timing, and extent of the trauma; and reactions to it.

CONCLUSIONS

When faced with trauma, the individual may go through stages of healing. The length of time, the intensity of emotions, and the outcomes are unique to that person. Factors such as resilience and adaptive/nonadaptive coping mechanisms impact how trauma is resolved. Posttraumatic growth is possible, which can bring a renewed sense of enthusiasm toward life, a compassion toward others, and a deeper purpose to guide decisions and actions. Individual strategies toward healing begin with recognition and acknowledgment that there is something that has happened to the individual. According to Buddhist philosophy, pain is unavoidable, but suffering is optional.

HIGHLIGHTS OF CHAPTER CONTENT

- According to Herman (2015), healing from trauma occurs in three stages (establishing safety, remembrance and mourning, and reconnecting with ordinary life).

- Resiliency may be viewed as a trait, a process, a defense mechanism, or an outcome, depending upon the context, the resources available, and the individual.

- Individual strategies discussed include: positive relationships and social support, journaling, mindfulness, mindfulness meditation, maintenance of daily structure and circadian rhythm, avoiding harmful self-medicating, human-animal bond, and finding purpose in life through psycho-spiritual transformation.

- Digital natives should be aware of how to evaluate apps designed to promote positive mental health.

- Specific therapies designed as treatment for adults, youth, and children affected by trauma may be found in the Evidence-Based Practices Resource Center (SAMHSA, 2018).

REFERENCES

American Psychiatric Association. (2013). *Diagnostic and statistical manual of mental disorders* (5th ed.). Arlington, VA: Author.

Asok, A., Bernard, K., Roth, T. L., Rosen, J. B., & Dozier, M. (2013). Parental responsiveness moderates the association between early-life stress and reduced telomere length. *Development and Psychopathology, 25*(3), 577–585. doi:10.1017/S0954579413000011

Beck, J. (2011). *Cognitive behavior therapy: Basics and beyond.* New York, NY: Guilford Press.

Borg, K. (2018). Narrating trauma: Judith Butler on narrative coherence and the politics of self-narration. *Life Writing, 15*(3), 447–465. doi:10.1080/14484528.2018.1475056

Bormann, J. E. (2014). Mantram repetition: A portable, mindful, contemplative practice for the workplace. *American Nurse Today, 9*(4), n.p.

Bormann, J. E., Hurst, S., & Kelly, A. (2013). Responses to mantram repetition program from veterans with posttraumatic stress disorder: A qualitative analysis. *Journal of Rehabilitation Research and Development, 50*(6), 769–784. doi:http://dx.doi.org/10.1682/JRRD.2012.06.0118

Bormann, J. E., Oman, D., Walter, K. H., & Johnson, B. D. (2014). Brief report: Mindful attention increases and mediates psychological outcomes following mantram repetition practice in veterans with posttraumatic stress disorder. *Medical Care, 52*(12), S13–S18.

Bormann, J. E., Thorp, S. R., Wetherell, J. L., Golshan, S., & Lang, A. J. (2013). Mediation-based mantram intervention for veterans with posttraumatic stress disorder: A randomized trial. *Psychological Trauma: Theory, Research, Practice, and Policy, 5*(3), 259–267.

Bray, P. (2010). A broader framework for exploring the influence of spiritual experience in the wake of stressful life events: Examining connections between posttraumatic growth and psycho-spiritual transformation. *Mental Health, Religion & Culture, 13*(3), 293–308. doi:10.1080/13674670903367199

Burnett, Jr., H. J. (2017). Revisiting the compassion fatigue, burnout, compassion satisfaction, and resilience connection among CISM responders. *Journal of Police Emergency Response/Sage Open*, 1–10. doi:10.1177/2158244017730857

Colman, A. M. (2015). Post-traumatic growth. In *A dictionary of psychology* (4th ed.). Oxford, UK: Oxford University Press.

Dekel, R. (2017). My personal and professional trauma resilience truisms. *Traumatology, 23*(1), 10–17. doi:http://dx.doi.org/10.1037/trm0000106

Evans, S. E., Steel, A. L., & DiLillo, D. (2013). Child maltreatment severity and adult trauma symptoms: Does perceived social support play a buffering role? *Child Abuse and Neglect, 37*, 934–943. doi:http://dx.doi.org/10.1016/j.chiabu.2013.03.005

Garcia-Dia, M. J., DiNapoli, J. M., Garcia-Ona, L., Jakubowski, R., & O'Flaherty, D. (2013). Concept analysis: Resilience. *Archives of Psychiatric Nursing, 27*, 264–270. doi:http://dx.doi.org/10.1016/j.apnu.2013.07.003

Herman, J. (2015). *Trauma and recovery: The aftermath of violence—From domestic abuse to political terror.* New York, NY: Basic Books.

Hevezi, J. A. (2016). Evaluation of a meditation intervention to reduce the effects of stressors associated with compassion fatigue among nurses. *Journal of Holistic Nursing, 34*(4), 343–350. doi:10.1177/0898010115615981

Hunter, A. J., & Chandler, G. E. (1999). Adolescent resilience. *Journal of Nursing Scholarship, 31*(3), 243–247.

Institute of Medicine. (2015). *Psychosocial interventions for mental and substance use disorders: A framework for establishing evidence-based standards.* Washington, DC: The National Academies Press.

Kabat-Zinn, J. (2015). Mindfulness. *Mindfulness, (6)*6, 1481–1483. doi:10.1007/s12671-015-0456-x

Kübler-Ross, E., & Kessler, D. (2014). *On grief & grieving: Finding the meaning of grief through the five stages of loss.* New York, NY: Scribner.

Li, Y., Cao, F., Cao, D., & Liu, J. (2015). Nursing students' post-traumatic growth, emotional intelligence and psychological resilience. *Journal of Psychiatric and Mental Health Nursing, 22*, 326–332. doi:10.1111/jpm.12192

Münzer, A., Ganser, H. G., & Goldbeck, L. (2017). Social support, negative maltreatment-related cognitions and posttraumatic stress symptoms in children and adolescents. *Child Abuse and Neglect, 63*, 183–191. doi:http://dx.doi.org/10.1016/j.chiabu.2016.11.015

Nightingale, F. (2009 ed.). *Notes on nursing.* New York, NY: Fall River Press.

Niitsu, K., Houfek, J. F., Barron, C. R., Stoltengerg, S. F., Kupzyk, K. A., & Rice, M. J. (2017). A concept analysis of resilience integrating genetics. *Issues in Mental Health Nursing, 38*(11), 896–906. doi:10.1080/01612840.2017.1350225

Panda, S. (2016). Circadian physiology of metabolism. *Science, 354*(6315), 1008–1015. doi:10.1126/science.aah4967

Pichot, T. (2013). *Animal-assisted brief therapy: A solution-focused approach* (2nd ed.). East Sussex, UK: Routledge.

Prensky, M. (2001). Digital natives, digital immigrants. *On the Horizon, 9*(5), 1–6. doi:10.1108/10748120110424816

PsyberGuide. (2018). About PsyberGuide. Retrieved from https://psyberguide.org/about-psyberguide/

Shapiro, F. (1995/2001). *Eye movement desensitization and reprocessing (EMDR) therapy: Basic principles, protocols, and procedures.* New York, NY: Guilford Press.

Substance Abuse and Mental Health Services Administration. (2014). Guiding principles of trauma-informed care. *SAMSHA News, 22*(2). Retrieved from https://www.samhsa.gov/samhsaNewsLetter/Volume_22_Number_2/trauma_tip/guiding_principles.html

Substance Abuse and Mental Health Services Administration. (2018). Evidence-based practices resource center. Retrieved from https://www.samhsa.gov/ebp-resource-center

Tedeschi, R. G., & Calhoun, L. G. (1995). *Trauma and transformation: Growing in the aftermath of suffering.* Thousand Oaks, CA: Sage.

Tedeschi, R. G., & Calhoun, L. G. (1996). The Posttraumatic Growth Inventory: Measuring the positive legacy of trauma. *Journal of Traumatic Stress, 9*(3), 455–471.

Tedeschi, R. G., & Calhoun, L. G. (2004). Target article: Posttraumatic growth: Conceptual foundations and empirical evidence. *Psychological Inquiry, 15*(1), 1–18. doi:10.1207/s15327965pli1501_01

Tedeschi, R. G., Cann, A., Taku, K., Senol-Durak, E., & Calhoun, L. G. (2017). The Posttraumatic Growth Inventory: A revision integrating existential and spiritual change. *Journal of Traumatic Stress, 30*, 11–18. doi:10.1002/jts

Turner, J. K., Hutchinson, A., & Wilson, C. (2018). Correlates of post-traumatic growth following childhood and adolescent cancer: A systematic review and meta-analysis. *Psycho-Oncology, 27*, 1100–1109. doi:10.1002/pon.4577

van der Rieta, P., Levett-Jones, T., & Aquino-Russell, C. (2018). The effectiveness of mindfulness meditation for nurses and nursing students: An integrated literature review. *Nursing Education Today, 65*, 201–211. doi:https://doi.org/10.1016/j.nedt.2018.03.018

van Wyk, M., Thomas, K. G., Solms, M., & Lipinska, G. (2016). Prominence of hyperarousal symptoms explains variability of sleep disruption in posttraumatic stress disorder. *Psychological Trauma: Theory, Research, Practice, and Policy, 8*(6), 688–696. doi:http://dx.doi.org/10.1037/tra0000115

Weinberg, M. (2017). Trauma and social support: The association between informal social support, formal social support, and psychological well-being among terror attack survivors. *International Social Work, 60*(1), 208–218. doi:https://doi-org.ezproxy.lib.purdue.edu/10.1177/0020872814564704

Wynn, G. H. (2015). Complementary and alternative medicine approaches in the treatment of PTSD. *Current Psychiatry Reports, 17*(8), 600. doi:10.1007/s11920-015-0600-2

Yoon, S. (2018). Fostering resilient development: Protective factors underlying externalizing trajectories of maltreated children. *Journal of Child and Family Studies, 27*, 443–452. doi:10.1007/s10826-017-0904-4

Young, S. (1994). Purpose and method of Vipassana meditation. *The Humanistic Psychologist, 22*(1), 53–61. doi:10.1080/08873267.1994.9976936

LEARNING OBJECTIVES

At the end of this chapter, you will be able to:

- Evaluate the need for the integration of trauma-informed competencies in nursing education.
- Critique the American Psychological Association's 2015 trauma competencies.
- Summarize that for the generalist nurse, trauma-informed care (TIC) spans multiple clinical areas (not confined to psychiatric-mental health nursing).
- Map the American Association of Colleges of Nursing's 2008 Essentials of Baccalaureate Education with TIC.
- Translate the Substance Abuse and Mental Health Services Administration's (SAMHSA's) trauma-informed care guiding principles to nursing work environments.
- Discuss aspects of psychological and physical safety in the workplace, including safe and reliable healthcare organizations, second-victim trauma, workplace violence, and nurses' substance use.
- Outline nursing supervisors' core competencies of secondary traumatic stress (STS).
- Theorize about the relationship between nurse retention and attachment to organizations.

TRAUMA-INFORMED PRACTICES IN EDUCATIONAL AND HEALTHCARE ORGANIZATIONS

5

PURPOSE OF THE CHAPTER

In this chapter, we move, temporarily, from the individual level to a larger context: the organization. We discuss both the student nurse and the new nurse embedded in institutions that should have trauma-informed practices and standards threaded into their culture and operations. As the largest health profession workforce, nurses often are hesitant about how and when to use their influence in organizations. Unfortunately, nurses are often subjected to traumatic events by being in organizations that do not recognize and safeguard them against vulnerabilities and harm. In the following discussion, we outline and discuss the trauma-informed standards, guidelines, and recommendations of educational and healthcare organizations. We hope in this way, you'll be supported as students and new nurses to better understand what practices trauma-informed systems should adhere to.

EDUCATIONAL COMPETENCIES IN TRAUMA-INFORMED CARE

The *Journal of the American Psychiatric Nurses Association* (2018) recently devoted an entire issue to trauma and trauma-informed care (TIC). In the guest editorial, Kathleen Wheeler called for nursing education to ensure that advanced practice nurses in psychiatric care and across all specialties, as well as undergraduate students, were prepared to render care that was trauma-competent. We heartily agree with Dr. Wheeler's call to action, and in this section, we provide an initial attempt to address competencies in student nurses who are preparing for initial licensure.

Such standards have been established for beginning psychologists. The American Psychological Association (2015) prepared aspirational and minimal competencies, which comprise knowledge, skills, and attitudes, for psychologists working with individuals with histories of trauma. Nine cross-cutting competencies, which included the impact of trauma and understanding reactions to trauma, were described. In addition to these, five core competencies were identified:

1. Scientific knowledge (for example, recognize epidemiology of trauma, various models, and cultural contexts)

2. Psychological assessment (inquire into trauma history and ability to perform a comprehensive assessment)

3. Psychological intervention (implement practices based on evidence, with individualization)

4. Professionalism (demonstrate legal and ethical awareness)

5. Relational and systems (interdisciplinary collaboration and delivery of content to audiences)

PSYCHIATRIC-MENTAL HEALTH NURSING: STANDARDS OF PRACTICE

In 2011, a task force made up of members from the American Psychiatric Nurses Association and the International Society of Psychiatric-Mental Health Nurses convened to update the psychiatric-mental health nursing scope and standards of practice. The result was an updated manual that outlines psychiatric-mental health nursing for both registered nurses and advanced practice nurses (American Nurses Association [ANA], 2014). Of note, trauma is cited numerous times within the standards framework of the nursing process: assessment, diagnosis, outcomes identification, planning, implementation, evaluation, and standards of professional performance (ANA, 2014). Trauma is a phenomenon of concern for psychiatric-mental health nurses, cutting across populations and life span and related to "alternation in self-concept" (ANA, 2014, p. 21). The standards also urge TIC and the reduction or the elimination of inducing new trauma through seclusion and restraint in various levels of care. Work is currently underway to create competencies for trauma and resilience in nursing education.

Although it is tempting to compartmentalize the effects of trauma and promote healing as a separate area of nursing, we need to resist this temptation. To adhere to and value the notion of holistic care, trauma is infused in all areas of nursing. Indeed, graduate students, who are returning to school for advanced practice degrees, will vigorously comment on how they never understood until beginning their practices how significant patients' mental health needs are. These are baccalaureate-prepared, generalist nurses who practice in a wide range of settings. In addition, there are nurses practicing at an advanced level who are educated and trained in psychiatric nursing to conduct therapy, prescribe medications, and manage care in groups of patients who have experienced trauma. For now, this chapter is for you, the generalist nurse who will see many patients across care settings and whose lives have been impacted by stressful, traumatic events.

NURSING EDUCATION: ESSENTIALS AND STANDARDS

Two organizations in nursing outline competency standards and essentials for nurses: The National League for Nursing and the American Association of Colleges of Nursing (AACN). Both influential organizations provide guidance for nursing educational content, accreditation, and standards for faculty at both the undergraduate and graduate levels. You may be a student in either an associate or a baccalaureate program or a new graduate from a program designed to prepare you for practice and pass the National Council Licensure Examination (NCLEX). But how do these essentials and standards link to trauma-informed nursing care?

In 2008, the AACN updated the nine baccalaureate essentials, ranging from standards and content from a foundation in the liberal arts, to leadership, to practice as a generalist in nursing. Each essential has a conceptual link with the delivery of compassionate, safe care related to nurses' TIC. In Table 5.1, we've offered the nine essentials (AACN, 2008) and created trauma-informed, sample content we believe is linked to the essential.

TABLE 5.1 THE AACN: ESSENTIALS OF BACCALAUREATE EDUCATION

ESSENTIAL	SAMPLE CONTENT RELATED TO TRAUMA-INFORMED CARE
Essential I: Liberal Education for Baccalaureate Generalist Nursing Practice	Exposure to natural science content to help the nurse understand the neurobiological/physiological changes that occur when an individual encounters trauma. Learning content from psychology and sociology describing trauma. Understanding cultural and social contexts of care.

Essential II: Basic Organizational and Systems Leadership for Quality Care and Patient Safety	Awareness of how organizations provide for employee safety and foster a healthy work environment. Emphasis that patient safety includes psychological perceptions of safety. Quality improvement projects that seek to strengthen patient care environments to lessen "treatment trauma."
Essential III: Scholarship for Evidence-Based Practice	Ability to apply theories surrounding trauma and symptomatology post trauma. Identification of empirical studies to support interventions with individuals exposed to trauma. Discrimination between anecdotal, theoretical, qualitative, and quantitative works that describe trauma in nursing care.
Essential IV: Information Management and Application of Patient Care Technology	Assurance that new technologies do not cause trauma and contribute instead to safety and patient control. Patient confidentiality, especially in disclosure of protected health information that is sensitive and, if shared inappropriately, could cause psychological trauma. Documentation in the health record identifies patient behaviors that may be explained within the trauma context.
Essential V: Health Care Policy, Finance, and Regulatory Environments	Policy at multiple levels that support individuals, groups, communities, and populations that have been affected by disasters, fleeing geographic spaces of harm and disadvantaged backgrounds. Support of processes that appropriately address second-victim trauma.
Essential VI: Interprofessional Communication and Collaboration for Improving Patient Health Outcomes	Actions to diminish lateral and horizontal violence (bullying, incivility, and so on) within nursing and across disciplines. Implementation of therapeutic communication with patients, peers, and colleagues. Inclusion of individuals as participants in their care, offering them respect and control.
Essential VII: Clinical Prevention and Population Health	Contribution to preparations for disaster management and recovery. Content on social determinants of health and the potential relationships between trauma and vulnerable groups. Inclusion of intergenerational trauma into health assessments.

continues

TABLE 5.1   THE AACN: ESSENTIALS OF BACCALAUREATE EDUCATION (CONT.)

Essential VIII: Professionalism and Professional Values	Understanding of the values inherent in nursing, including protecting human dignity for those experiencing trauma. Self-awareness of implicit and explicit biases and how these may affect care (mitigate or cause trauma). Involvement in self-care to process secondary trauma and prevent compassion fatigue.
Essential IX: Baccalaureate Generalist Nursing Practice	Performance of assessments, arrival at nursing diagnoses, intervention planning, and evaluation of care with an awareness of the patient who has experienced trauma. Provision of education to individuals knowing that their readiness to learn content, adhere to treatment plans, and internalize goals will be affected by trauma experiences. Spiritual care with sensitivity toward the ability of the individual to forgive and process loss.

Source: AACN, 2008

PRINCIPLES OF TRAUMA-INFORMED CARE FOR NURSES IN ORGANIZATIONS

Today, we know about effective, evidence-based interventions for individuals who have experienced trauma, along with organizations that support TIC. The nearby sidebar offers six guiding principles outlined by SAMHSA (2014) that describe how the ecosystem of organization, staff, and clients exist in a trauma-informed environment. As described previously, individuals need to feel safe. As we now understand, those who have experienced trauma crave the feeling of safety. In the clinical setting, we as nurses hold nonjudgmental acceptance of illness states and individual cultural and spiritual preferences in high regard. Their brains need to pause, rest, and break the flight, fight, and freeze reactions.

The feeling of safety isn't confined to those who seek services. The staff within the organization must also feel a sense of physical and psychological safety (SAMHSA, 2014). In the educational setting, this translates to an allowance of human error with accountability, civility, and students being treated equally by faculty. We exercised intellectual freedom by translating SAMHSA's six guiding principles of trauma-informed care to standards specific to nurses working in organizations.

SAMHSA'S SIX GUIDING PRINCIPLES OF TRAUMA-INFORMED CARE

Principle 1: Safety

Principle 2: Trustworthiness and transparency

Principle 3: Peer support and mutual self-help

Principle 4: Collaboration and mutuality

Principle 5: Empowerment, voice, and choice

Principle 6: Cultural, historical, and gender issues

Source: SAMHSA, 2014

PRINCIPLE 1: TO FEEL SAFE, A NURSE NEEDS ADEQUATE RESOURCES, INCLUDING STAFFING LEVELS, TO PROVIDE QUALITY CARE.

Safety is not only about patient outcomes, which may be impacted by the lack of quality care. It is also about safe staffing levels and the stress nurses experience from an inability to meet patients' needs because there simply aren't enough nurses to competently care for those who need them. The ANA (2015) endorses flexible staffing based on transparency of organizations in determining staffing ratios. Public data reflecting staffing should be provided, and optimal nursing staffing should consider:

> patient complexity, acuity, or stability; number of admissions, discharges, and transfers; professional nursing and other staff skill level and expertise; physical space and layout of the nursing unit; and availability of or proximity to technological support or other resources. (ANA, 2015, p. 4)

Evidence also supports the value in human/staff, economic, and patient outcomes. The ANA (2015) further states that when federal guidance is issued, penalties should be in place for organizations that do not comply. Shortsightedness in healthcare organizations that do not appreciate the evidence to support optimal staffing seems to have exposed several groups to psychological trauma: the nurse who knows he cannot meet the patient's needs and is fearful harm will be done; professionals who collaborate with nursing whose treatment plan is not implemented; and the patient whose care is substandard due to inadequate nursing care.

Another effect of short staffing is on current employees: requests for overtime with longer hours and additional shifts. These practices result in nurses becoming fatigued with disrupted circadian rhythms. We understand nurse fatigue has a negative impact on patient safety and nurse well-being. An additional contributor to nurse fatigue is frequent shift rotations, which again can contribute to disruptions in circadian rhythms. The American Academy of Nursing (AAN), through the Health Behavior Expert Panel (Caruso et al., 2017), issued a position statement that urged nurses and healthcare organization leaders to implement ways to prevent nurse fatigue and foster a safe environment. The AAN's panel recommended: educating on nurse fatigue and health risks, using evidence-based practice when designing nurse shifts and work hours, fostering a culture of sleep health, recognizing negative outcomes resulting from nurse fatigue, and creating continuing education for nurses to "maximize sleep health and alertness in nurses" (Caruso et al., 2017, p. 767).

PRINCIPLE 2: TO TRUST, NURSES HAVE TO BELIEVE THAT THEIR VOICES ARE HEARD IN AN ORGANIZATION, WHICH IS TRANSPARENT IN ITS POLICIES TO SUPPORT NURSING STAFF.

Often when trauma occurs, there is a breach of trust. Within the organization, *shared governance,* a working relationship between leadership, middle managers, and front-line workers, adds to a feeling of reliability and dependability. Transparency of organizational mission, decision-making, and procedures facilitates nurses' trust. Similarly, as quality improvement projects are implemented, nurses' ideal state solutions and strategies toward ensuring sustainability need acted upon.

PRINCIPLE 3: SUPERVISORS AND PEERS ARE CIVIL WITH EACH OTHER, FOSTER RESPECT, AND BUILD ONE ANOTHER UP THROUGH SHARED LIVED EXPERIENCES.

Supervisor and peer assistance extend effective support to nurses. These values stem from authentic and servant leaders who understand that empowering those who provide services can positively impact the milieu. Multiple studies have reinforced the idea that social support is an important buffer to us as human beings. This is especially the case when individuals are in environments, such as healthcare, which are infused with firsthand and secondary trauma. Nurses bond and use humor to offset stress; nursing units with low turnover rates are often those where nurses ensure the welfare of one another. In addition, the literature describing being a good follower in an organization is growing. The stress on supervisors and managers is intense in most healthcare facilities, and being a trusted follower who understands psychological safety is an asset.

PRINCIPLE 4: NURSES COLLABORATE WITH EACH OTHER AND OTHER PROFESSIONS THROUGH RECIPROCITY IN SHARING RESOURCES, TALENT, AND TIME. THERE IS ZERO TOLERANCE FOR BULLYING.

Consider the trauma that can be avoided when people help each other. They know they are viewed as unique human beings with different talents, strengths, and challenges. The challenges of each individual are accepted, and opportunities for growth in these areas are part of no-risk development plans. In addition, interprofessional communication is enhanced. Those with power don't abuse it and, in fact, demonstrate compassion toward team members.

PRINCIPLE 5: SELF-GOVERNANCE IS EMBEDDED IN THE ORGANIZATION AND PROTECTED BY THE CHIEF NURSING OFFICER, WHO ENSURES NURSES ACTING AS "FRONT-LINE" SERVICE PROVIDERS HAVE A VOICE IN DECISIONS.

We have heard from nurses, who present as beginning graduate students, remark that some of their motivation to become advanced practitioners is bred from a lack of voice as a bedside nurse. Self-governance was in "name only." They want to become more independent, and therefore, more able to control their environments. Feeling helpless can certainly lead to feeling unsafe, and without a voice to affect needed change, nurses are apt to leave those organizations or even the profession. Top management should actively solicit point-of-service providers' feedback, at times without this information being filtered through middle managers.

Leadership at the top can be rewarding: highly visible positions that include significant formal authority. Along with the perks come responsibilities to ensure that those who depend upon their leadership (not management of resources alone) will be able to trust in them. Managerial risk can make a person feel unsafe, but on occasion, it is what separates a complacent leader from a visionary. Willingness to accept risk and even ridicule on behalf of those who are being served is the mark of a brave leader.

PRINCIPLE 6: MULTIFACETED CONTEXTS, INCLUDING CULTURE, HISTORY, GENDER, IMPLICIT BIASES, AND SOCIAL DETERMINANTS, ARE RECOGNIZED.

Organizations become communities, essentially their own ecosystems, where people spend the majority of their time. Missions and philosophies influence the worth of the brand internally and externally. As such, respect and safety for nurses' diversity, equity, and culture within the organization harbors a trauma-informed approach. This can stem from an authentic organizational culture where the truth is spoken, moral self-awareness is facilitated, and courage is rewarded.

PSYCHOLOGICAL SAFETY WITHIN ORGANIZATIONS

In Chapter 2, we discussed the phenomenon of second-victim trauma, trauma that occurs as a result of an error made by a nurse/healthcare professional. The name captures a "first" victim, the patient who has been impacted by the error, and the "second" victim, the provider who made the error. One organization, now with an increasingly global focus, has forwarded ways to improve healthcare quality: the Institute for Healthcare Improvement (IHI), officially founded in 1991 (IHI, 2018). The mission of this organization is to "improve health and healthcare worldwide" (IHI, 2018, "Our Mission"). We often equate patient safety to the avoidance and reduction of errors during care delivery.

Interestingly, the IHI is also talking about *psychological* safety. In its "Framework for Safe, Reliable, and Effective Care" (Frankel, Haraden, Federico, & Lenoci-Edwards, 2017), nine components are described:

1. Leadership

2. Psychological safety

3. Accountability

4. Teamwork and communication

5. Negotiation

6. Transparency

7. Reliability

8. Improvement and measurement

9. Continuous learning

Of note is that the second component is psychological safety. Frankel et al. (2017) describe psychological safety as the ability of any party within a healthcare organization, including patients, families, and staff, to voice opinions, concerns, and feedback in a safe environment. Concerns of retaliation or feeling "stupid" or being perceived as negative, incompetent, or disruptive are absent (Frankel et al., 2017, p. 11). A flat hierarchy, hearing people's ideas without judgment and allowing for those ideas that organically arise during brainstorming, helps to foster a milieu of safety (Frankel et al., 2017, p. 11). As individuals feel safe to articulate perceptions and information, the organization's delivery of care will, in turn, be safer.

Organizations are also addressing second victims' emotional needs. One model used by Johns Hopkins Hospital is Resilience in Stressful Events (RISE; Edrees et al., 2016). In this approach, RISE is used to address the needs of healthcare providers who have experienced adverse events. The model supplements the traditional method of reporting an adverse event or medical error, which typically entails reporting the event to the manager with a corresponding incident report. As a peer-support program, RISE uses an on-call paging system to respond to providers when adverse events occur (for example, medical errors, patient deaths, burnout, and staff assault). Interactions between the second victim and responder are confidential (excluding reports of self-harm). Edrees et al. (2016) report that responders' perceptions of the RISE program, from January 2010 to June 2012, reveal that most responders rated the success of the interactions as excellent (66.7%). Interestingly, registered nurses made most of the calls to responders (Edrees et al., 2016).

NURSES WITH DISABILITIES

Having a disability, whether physical or mental, can be stigmatizing and traumatizing. While organizational policies vary, we want to draw attention to accommodations for student nurses and nurses with disabilities in schools and in the workforce. Authors such as Donna Carol Maheady have written extensively on supporting nurses with disabilities entering the workplace. Organizations also advocate for nurses with disabilities and include the National Organization of Nurses with Disabilities (n.d.) and Exceptional Nurse, founded by Maheady (2011).

PREVENTING WORKPLACE VIOLENCE FOR NURSES

The National Institute for Occupational Safety and Health (NIOSH) offers a free online course to assist nurses in preventing workplace violence (NIOSH, 2016). Modules within the course include the definition of workplace violence, consequences of workplace violence, risk factors, prevention strategies, interventions strategies, and case studies. Several clinical contexts are offered, such as psychiatric patients in the ED, homicidal patients in home care, and inappropriate sexual behaviors exhibited by patients (NIOSH, 2016). Being aware of nonverbal communication and being attuned to the environment are two techniques offered in this 13-unit online course.

SUBSTANCE USE IN NURSING

Substance use disorders (SUDs) in nursing is an underdeveloped area of research, and in the practice setting, it blurs legal and ethical realms. The issue we face is, where do we situate nurses who have SUDs? Do we place them in the legal/criminal justice system because often laws are broken? Or should we frame them as individuals with a medical disease, impacting both mental and physical health? We know that SUDs experienced by nurses present safety issues for the individual and for the public. When a nurse is practicing in an impaired state, peers may have picked up on cues, but because of various reasons, decided to ignore those signs. However, those signs may not be obvious. Nurses who use substances may be the overachievers on the units, the ones who win awards, and the ones who volunteer to work extra shifts. When diversion or use is discovered, supervisors and peers are surprised, disappointed, and dismayed to learn their colleague is impaired.

For some nurses, a trigger leads to the misuse of substances, the diversion of drugs, and ultimately, dependence. Such a trigger may stem from physical or psychological trauma: a physical injury that requires pain medication or overwhelming secondary trauma that has been endured for years. Regardless of why the nurse begins to use substances, one of the priority areas of the National Council of State Boards of Nursing (NCSBN, 2018a), an independent, not-for-profit organization with a mission to support regulatory excellence in nursing, is substance use in nurses. This organization has taken the lead on developing and disseminating toolkits, free continuing education materials, and manuals to assist nurses and nursing supervisors. (See ncsbn.org/sud-nursing [NCSBN, 2018b] to access these resources.)

Alternative-to-discipline programs provide mechanisms for nurses to self-report SUDs, which may positively impact the disciplinary actions taken by the state board of nursing (Russell, 2017). The nurse agrees to a recovery monitoring agreement, which often requires random drug screens, supervisor reports (if license is not suspended), and check-ins with the program administrators/counselors. In a qualitative study of administrators, supervisors, and managers who interact with nurses in recovery and re-entering the workplace, researchers describe compassion and a show of personal values in welcoming the nurse back into the organization (Miller, Kanai, Kebritch, Grendell, & Howard, 2015). We hope that nurses' recovery efforts are situated in caring, balanced with accountability, to facilitate a life free from substance dependency.

THE NURSING SUPERVISOR

Perhaps you've always wanted to lead others. Or you believe your efforts could have a broader influence through directing services delivered by supervised individuals. There may have been someone who has led with authenticity and competence in your life whom you aspire to emulate. Marrying the two—authentic leadership and trauma-informed principles—is what the National Child Traumatic Stress Network (2018) has prepared in the "Secondary Trauma Stress (STS)—Core Competencies for Supervisors" (see the nearby sidebar). In these nine competencies, supervisors are charged with having the knowledge and skills to guide and mentor staff members who may be exposed to trauma, experience secondary trauma stress, or feel compassion fatigue.

Insight into themselves and their own processing of such trauma are key to being available to staff. Being fearless, as well as thoughtful and skillful, in coaching and addressing secondary trauma stress is needed. Having conversations in an environment of safety allows an exchange that has the potential to begin the process of healing the caregiver so that the caregiver, in turn, can deliver optimal care to patients.

SECONDARY TRAUMA STRESS (STS)—CORE COMPETENCIES FOR SUPERVISORS

1. Knowledge of the signs, symptoms, and risk factors of STS and its impact on employees; knowledge of agency support options, referral process for employee assistance, or external support resources for supervisees who are experiencing symptoms of STS.

2. Knowledge and capacity to self-assess, monitor, and address the supervisor's personal STS.

3. Knowledge of how to encourage employees in sharing the emotional experience of doing trauma work in a safe and supportive manner.

4. Skills to assist the employee in emotional re-regulation after difficult encounters; capacity to assess the effectiveness of intervention, monitor progress and make appropriate referrals, if necessary.

5. Knowledge of basic Psychological First Aid (PFA) or other supportive approaches to assist staff after an emergency or crisis event.

6. Ability to both model and coach supervisees in using a trauma lens to guide case conceptualization and service delivery.

7. Knowledge of resiliency factors and ability to structure resilience-building into individual and group supervisory activities.

8. Ability to distinguish between expected changes in supervisee perspectives and cognitive distortions related to indirect trauma exposure.

9. Ability to use appropriate self-disclosure in supervisory sessions to enhance the supervisee's ability to recognize, acknowledge, and respond to the impact of indirect trauma.

Source: National Child Traumatic Stress Network, 2018

We believe that good leaders are in short supply. The market pressures on patient care, the emphasis on technology, and the intensity of patient acuity create a risk-averse environment where speaking out against the dominant paradigm represents negative consequences for both a specific position and a career. Yet, we also believe that a good leader has the ability to positively affect careers, increase a sense of community, and decrease the aftermath of traumas.

NURSE RETENTION AND ATTACHMENT

Nurse retention is part of the issue when the nursing shortage is discussed. And there is no question: We are facing a nursing shortage. The population is aging, healthcare is becoming more complex, and there is a shortage of nursing faculty to teach. Compounding the shortage is nurse turnover, which may be across organizations or those who choose to leave the profession altogether. Those nurses who elect to leave an organization or the profession do so for a number of reasons.

As we've noted in Chapters 1 and 3, an important element in trauma is attachment; individuals may lack trust in others and have difficulty attaching. We are curious to know whether this extends to organizations that, through misguided policies and staffing levels, have been places of trauma for nurses. Thus, do these trauma-inducing spaces also affect an employee (nurse), their attachment to the organization, and ultimately, the decision to leave (either the healthcare organization or the profession)?

A report written by lead investigator Christine Kovner and the Robert Wood Johnson Foundation (RWJF, 2013) describes the areas that influence whether new nurses leave an organization. Factors surrounding retention include: opportunities for professional growth and promotion (for example, nurses want to know there is upward expansion), organizational constraints (not enough supplies to do their work), decision-making procedures and autonomy (for example, fairness and involvement in decisions), and poor quality nurse management (RWJF, 2013).

We ask whether these items equate to organizational commitment as a proxy for attachment to an organization in relation to intention to leave. Organizational commitment and job satisfaction have been shown to have an indirect effect on intention to stay in an organization (Brewer, Chao, Colder, Kovner, & Chacko, 2015). We recommend more research be conducted into the role of organizational trauma, attachment/commitment, and nurse retention.

We would be remiss to omit the work that has been accomplished by the American Association of Critical-Care Nurses (2016), which established six essential standards for a healthy work environment: skilled communication, true collaboration, effective decision-making, appropriate staffing, meaningful recognition, and authentic leadership. Several of these standards can be linked to a nurse's attachment to peers and organizations. For example, true collaboration means that partnerships are more than "lip service" to decision-making. The reciprocal relationship means that everyone is respected, and roles are differentiated in an appropriate way. Recognition means those who know how to "market themselves" aren't the only ones being called out for excellence in performance.

To emphasize the global nature of the workplace, the World Health Organization (WHO) describes four "avenues for a healthy workplace" (Burton, 2010, p. 83). These are: 1) the physical work environment; 2) the psychosocial work environment; 3) personal health resources in the workplace; and 4) enterprise community involvement (Burton, 2010, p. 83). Here, we discuss the second avenue, the psychosocial environment, which includes how work is organized, the work culture, and practices, attitudes, beliefs, and values that affect the well-being of the worker. The WHO (Burton, 2010) also refers to these as workplace stressors. To address and alleviate these stressors, the WHO (Burton, 2010) recommends eliminating or modifying the source of the stress (for example, decrease workload, zero tolerance for harassment or bullying); lessening the impact on the employee (for example, allow flexibility and open communication); and protecting the worker (for example, train workers on stress management and conflict management techniques). The list is applicable across nations and cultures.

TRAUMA-INFORMED REFLECTION

Think about a recent clinical experience you had or, if you're a practicing nurse, a recent shift you worked. Did you assess a feeling of attachment from the staff to colleagues, to the interprofessional team, to the patients? How did this relate to the culture of the organization? Are these two constructs positively related? Do you think the attachment felt by the nurse is a predictor of her staying in the organization? In the profession of nursing? Why or why not?

CONCLUSIONS

Trauma-informed educational competencies should be infused and adapted to specific courses across the generalist nursing curricula. One way of infusing these competencies is via the AACN's (2008) Essentials of Baccalaureate Education. Healthcare organizations, nursing leaders, and nursing supervisors (middle managers) have a responsibility to foster psychological and physical safety of all workers, but with particular attention and resources given to nurses, who are at the point-of-service contact. Special populations of nurses, such as individuals with disabilities and substance use issues, should be integrated into organizations by balancing nurse, patient, and public safety factors.

HIGHLIGHTS OF CHAPTER CONTENT

- Principles of trauma-informed care should be infused in educational institutions as competencies and in healthcare organizations as standards of practice.

- In healthcare organizations, feelings of safety, competency, and trust are affected by staffing patterns, self-governance (participatory management), civility, deference to point-of-service providers, and respect for heterogeneity, including those with disabilities.

- Organizations may be the source or location of trauma for nurses; these include second-victim trauma and workplace violence.

- Nursing supervisors are integral to recognizing and mitigating secondary trauma stress of those working under their guidance, as well as creating a culture that facilitates attachment to the organization.

REFERENCES

American Association of Colleges of Nursing. (2008). *The essentials of baccalaureate education for professional nursing practice.* Washington, DC: Author.

American Association of Critical-Care Nurses. (2016). *AACN standards for establishing and sustaining healthy work environments: A journey to excellence* (2nd ed.). Aliso Viejo, CA: Author.

American Nurses Association. (2014). *Psychiatric-mental health nursing: Scope and standards of practice.* Silver Springs, MD: Author.

American Nurses Association. (2015). *Optimal nurse staffing to improve quality of care and patient outcomes: Executive summary.* Washington, DC: Author.

American Psychological Association. (2015). *Guidelines on trauma competencies for education and training.* Retrieved from http://www.apa.org/ed/resources/trauma-competencies-training.pdf

Brewer, C. S., Chao, Y-Y., Colder, C. R., Kovner, C. T., & Chacko, T. P. (2015). A structural equation model of turnover for a longitudinal survey among early career registered nurses. *International Journal of Nursing Studies, 52,* 1735–1745. doi:http.//dx.doi/org/10.1016/j.ijnurstu.2015.06.017

Burton, J. (2010). *WHO healthy workplace framework and model: Background and supporting literature and practices.* Geneva, Switzerland: World Health Organization. Retrieved from http://www.who.int/occupational_health/healthy_workplace_framework.pdf

Caruso, C. C., Baldwin, C. M., Berger, A., Chasens, E. R., Landis, C., Redeker, N. S., . . . Trinkoff, A. (2017). Position statement: Reducing fatigue associated with sleep deficiency and work hours in nurses. *Nursing Outlook, 65*(6), 766–768. doi:https://doi.org/10.1016/j.outlook.2017.10.011

Edrees, H., Connors, C., Paine, L., Norvell, M., Taylor, H., & Wu, A. W. (2016). Implementing the RISE second victim support programme at the Johns Hopkins Hospital: A case study. *British Medical Journal Open, 6,* 1–11. doi:10.1136/bmjopen-2016-011708

Exceptional Nurse. (2011). About ExceptionalNurse.com. Retrieved from http://www.exceptionalnurse.com/aboutus.php

Frankel, A., Haraden, C., Federico, F., & Lenoci-Edwards, J. A. (2017). *Framework for safe, reliable, and effective care* [White paper]. Cambridge, MA: Institute for Healthcare Improvement and Safe & Reliable Healthcare.

Institute for Healthcare Improvement. (2018). About us. Retrieved from http://www.ihi.org/about/Pages/IHIVisionandValues.aspx

Journal of the American Psychiatric Nurses Association. (January/February 2018). Focus issue on trauma. *24*(1).

Miller, T., Kanai, T., Kebritch, M., Grendell, R., & Howard, T. (2015). Hiring nurses re-entering the workforce after chemical dependence. *Journal of Nursing Education and Practice, 5*(11), 65–72. doi:10.5430/jnep.v5n11p65

National Child Traumatic Stress Network. (2018). *Using the Secondary Traumatic Stress Core Competencies in trauma-informed supervision.* Retrieved from https://www.nctsn.org/sites/default/files/resources/fact-sheet/using_the_secondary_traumatic_stress_core_competencies_in_trauma-informed_supervision.pdf

National Council of State Boards of Nursing. (2018a). About NCSBN. Retrieved from https://www.ncsbn.org/about.htm

National Council of State Boards of Nursing. (2018b). Substance use disorder in nursing. Retrieved from https://ncsbn.org/substance-use-in-nursing.htm

National Institute for Occupational Safety and Health. (2016). *Workplace violence prevention for nurses* [Online course]. Retrieved from https://wwwn.cdc.gov/wpvhc/Course.aspx/Slide/Intro_2

National Organization of Nurses with Disabilities. (n.d.). Who we are. Retrieved from https://nond.org/who-we-are/

Robert Wood Johnson Foundation. (2013). *The RN work project: A national study to track career changes among newly licensed registered nurses.* Retrieved from https://www.rwjf.org/content/dam/farm/reports/program_results_reports/2013/rwjf408872

Russell, K. A. (2017). Nurse practice acts guide and govern: Update 2017. *Journal of Nursing Regulation, 8*(3), 18–25.

Substance Abuse and Mental Health Services Administration. (Spring 2014). Guiding principles of trauma-informed care. *SAMSHA News, 22*(2). Retrieved from https://www.samhsa.gov/samhsaNewsLetter/Volume_22_Number_2/trauma_tip/guiding_principles.html

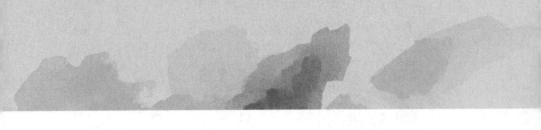

LEARNING OBJECTIVES

At the end of this chapter, you will be able to:

- Provide rationale for why nurses should apply trauma-informed care (TIC).

- Describe compassion, compassion satisfaction, self-compassion, team-based compassion, and the emancipatory theory of compassion (Georges, 2011, 2013).

- Reframe patient adherence within a paradigm of TIC.

- Map the ways of knowing (Carper, 1978; Chinn & Kramer, 2015) by applying TIC in a case study.

- Compare three theories that provide conceptualization and organizing frameworks that you can apply to TIC.

- Appraise the contributions of Mental Health First Aid and Psychological First Aid to TIC.

APPLYING TRAUMA-INFORMED CARE AS A NEW NURSE

6

PURPOSE OF THE CHAPTER

In this chapter, we discuss how to apply your newly found understanding and knowledge of trauma and bring it into the clinical setting. You began to appreciate different modalities of healing from trauma in Chapter 4—modalities at an individual level. In Chapter 5, we shifted our focus to concentrate on educational institutions and healthcare organizations and how trauma-informed practices should be infused into their cultures, competencies, and standards. In this chapter, we describe trauma-informed nursing care delivery, and within an organizational context specific to you, the practicing student/newly licensed nurse. The standing tenet of our discussion is that our care should always be trauma informed, regardless of the clinical setting or even an awareness of the patient's history. In the final analysis, implementing these principles, even in the absence of trauma, can be comforting and compassionate.

TRAUMA-INFORMED CARE IN NURSING: EVIDENCE FOR CHANGE

We view trauma-informed care (TIC) as part of competent nursing care. TIC is beginning to be viewed as an approach to all patients in any health-care context, not just mental health. Trauma is a universal experience; either ourselves or those we care about will face trauma at some point. But there is an art to this understanding, as well as principles to follow. Trauma-informed practices may stand in juxtaposition to existing practices that conflict with psychological safety, competency, and connections.

To gain an awareness of nurses' perceptions of TIC, Stokes, Jacob, Gifford, Squires, and Vandyk (2017) explore themes derived from semi-structured interviews with seven nurses who worked in mental health. One interesting theme was the "dynamics of the nurse-patient relationship in the face of trauma" (Stokes et al., 2017, p. 6). The authors describe how nurses may traumatize/retraumatize patients and, in a dynamic way, traumatize the nurses (secondary trauma). An additional theme, "Context of TIC," explores how TIC was more than checking a box to assess for trauma: Participants saw nurses performing duties in a set pattern, which they believed was an adverse practice in the context of TIC (Stokes et al., 2017, pp. 5–6). Included in this theme were the ideas of time being a barrier to exploration of trauma-informed practices, but also the value of integrating TIC in curricula and practice (Stokes et al., 2017).

At present, one of the limitations of TIC is how to translate best practices into daily nursing care. In a study by Isobel and Delgado (2018), an eight-hour workshop offered to 73 mental health nurses across 10 workshops was described. These workshops contained two role-playing simulations with one moderate- and one high-distress patient. Field notes reported by Isobel and Delgado (2018) describe how nurses were initially uncomfortable with role-playing and obtaining peer feedback within the context of TIC. Theoretical content for the workshop included environmental and group safety, what helps and hinders safety, and communication skills. Of note, one practical communication skill was "minimizing the use of 'no'" (p. 292). Ultimately, the nurses reported insight into their own practices. Some nurses were quick to skip to problem-solving, and the majority reported that the workshop impacted their practice and under-standing of TIC (Isobel & Delgado, 2018).

Within the acute psychiatric setting, seclusion and restraint are trauma-inducing events for both the patient and the caregiver. The Cen-ters for Medicare and Medicaid Services and the Joint Commission have implemented strict guidance on when seclusion and/or restraint should be used. The Substance Abuse and Mental Health Services Administra-tion (SAMHSA) is committed to eliminating the use of these measures for individuals with mental health issues. In a retrospective study, Azeem, Aujla, Rammerth, Binsfeld, and Jones (2011) found that by integrating trauma-informed principles, seclusion and restraints in an acute psychiat-ric hospital declined. The first six months of the study showed 93 seclu-sion/restraint episodes, whereas the last six months of the study, after staff training based on trauma-informed core strategies, showed 31 episodes. Interestingly, a core strategy used by the hospital, "Leadership Toward Organizational Change," prioritized a decrease in seclusion and restraints. Leaders operationalized this priority through a shared vision, training, and frequent communications, practices inherent in TIC (Azeem et al., 2011, p. 12).

General guidelines for interventions related to posttraumatic events are helpful as specific interventions are planned (SAMHSA, 2018; also see the "Trauma-Specific Interventions" sidebar). As programs are designed and implemented, the survivor's needs are listed first; this intentional place-ment emphasizes the individual being at the center of care. The second statement recognizes that the event or source of trauma creates symptoms. Healing is facilitated as the interplay between trauma occurrence and symptoms is uncovered, acknowledged, and worked through. In other words, the event creates ripples into the person's life (for example, mal-adaptive behaviors and distorted perceptions), and if we miss those ripples and only look at the stone that has been cast to cause the disruption, our efforts will be limited. In turn, when we only see the disruption of life caused by symptoms, we may not have unearthed the heart of the injury.

The last intervention guideline describes the necessity for collabora-tion between the social networks surrounding the individual who has been affected by trauma. These networks may be the agencies providing services, the circle of friends and family surrounding the individual, and supportive people who may have experienced similar trauma. When we share our trauma secrets with others, we expand our networks.

TRAUMA-SPECIFIC INTERVENTIONS

Trauma-specific intervention programs generally recognize the following:

- The survivor's need to be respected, informed, connected, and hopeful regarding her own recovery
- The interrelation between trauma and symptoms of trauma, such as substance abuse, eating disorders, depression, and anxiety
- The need to work in a collaborative way with survivors, family and friends of the survivor, and other human services agencies in a manner that empowers survivors and consumers

Source: SAMHSA, 2018

ADHERENCE

One factor that often impacts our ability to demonstrate compassionate care is when we become aware of treatment or medication adherence issues. Individuals who do not follow a plan of care often create care-giver frustration, annoyance, and impatience. This assumes a hierarchical relationship rather than a collaboration or partnership. To be compassionate when we consider adherence, we again need to be reminded of the psychological needs of those who have experienced trauma, including the need for safety, control, attachment, and emotional regulation.

When administering care to individuals, we have to respect the individual's need to feel safe. Promises may be difficult to keep, but acknowledgments can be offered. For example, a dressing change may be painful, and promising to keep a patient pain-free may not be realistic. However, acknowledging you are aware of the need for pain control and will act on this nursing intervention will help the patient feel more in control.

Decision-making during nursing care tasks is important. If a conversation about the care needs to happen in a nursing shift, offering options of how and when interventions are implemented supports the individual in sensing some control. To have adherence to treatment, the patient also must perceive a health threat's severity and barriers to care. Many theories explain how decisions involving health behaviors are formed. Two of the more prominent ones are the Health Belief Model (Rosenstock, Strecher, & Becker, 1988) and the Theory of Reasoned Action (Fishbein, 2008; Fishbein & Ajzen, 1975). Both of these models examine what the individual perceives about the health threat and how important the threat or disease is to them. When we examine how health behavior decisions are made, we may not account for the influence of trauma, which may, in turn, affect such constructs as subjective norms, self-efficacy, and motivation to comply.

We speak to many nurses who share how relationships are formed with patients in a variety of settings, including long-term care, pediatrics, primary care, and acute care. We become attached to them, and they become attached to us. Often in healthcare, patients are vulnerable and in crisis. The nurse-patient relationships may form quickly, organically, and authentically. The nurse who is trauma-informed will realize that relationships for those with a history of trauma may require more trust and more time and be subjected to continual testing. Their emotions may be labile and present unevenly, especially in the presence of trauma triggers or intrusive thoughts.

Emotional dysregulation, which may heighten during health crises or when facing chronic diseases over a long period of time, also affects adherence. We discussed the impact on development and the brain in Chapter 1; thus, nurses' goals should be imparting a sense of competency and safety, of nonjudgment and patience as they try to understand their patient's world that has been impacted by traumatic events.

COMPASSION: TYPES AND CONTEXTS

One closely aligned approach to implementing TIC is choosing to demonstrate compassion and use compassionate communication. We discussed compassion fatigue in Chapter 2; here we seek to define what compassion is and how compassion is extended to the self, to patients, and to the interprofessional team. Several concept analyses help illuminate the importance of compassion within the context of TIC.

The first concept analysis, published in 2007, began the conversations related to compassion in nursing (Schantz). It described compassion toward patients as a choice to apply a virtue inherent in human beings (Schantz, 2007). There is the antecedent of suffering, which must be identified and acknowledged for compassion to exist (Schantz, 2007). A similar concept that focuses on the nurse rather than the patient—compassion satisfaction—has been more recently developed. Compassion satisfaction rises from compassionate nursing interactions with patients and nurses (Mason & Nel, 2012).

The second concept analysis of compassion satisfaction by Sacco and Copel (2018) lists 11 feelings the nurse may experience in compassion satisfaction, including well-being, fulfillment, reward, accomplishment, and joy. Compassion satisfaction is viewed as potential protection to compassion fatigue. The authors define compassion satisfaction as: "the pleasure, purpose, and gratification received by professional caregivers through their contributions to the well-being of patients and their families" (Sacco & Copel, 2018, p. 78).

In addition to compassion satisfaction, there is a concept of "self-compassion" described by Reyes (2012). In this concept analysis, Reyes (2012) posits that the antecedent of self-compassion is suffering (similar to Schantz, 2007), and the characteristics that define self-compassion are self-kindness, mindfulness, common humanity, and wisdom. We find this analysis appropriate to our discussion of trauma. For example, self-kindness involves forgiveness of self for transgressions toward others. Common humanity refers to the individual acknowledging that his experiences are part of the larger humanity, creating a sense of community and belonging, versus isolation (Reyes, 2012). Thus, the themes of pain, recovery through wisdom, connections with others through a sense of common humanity, and awareness of the present have links to trauma recovery.

Compassion toward team members is another aspect to this concept. In a grounded theory study that examined qualitative data from 50 individuals involved in interviews and focus groups, researchers identified four characteristics of nurses' professional communication in teams:

collaboration, credibility, compassion, and coordination (Apker, Propp, Zabava Ford, & Hofmeister, 2006). Compassion encompassed showing respect and affiliation, advocating for other team members' concerns, and demonstrating consideration and caring toward others (Apker et al., 2006). Peer debriefing after trauma induced by care delivery is an example of how team-based compassion may ease us into healing. Being able to process events and emotions with those we work with in both formal and informal ways supports strong teams. Again, trauma-based themes are apparent when considering team interactions marked by compassion: feeling safe and fostering connections with others.

PATIENTS' PERSPECTIVES OF COMPASSIONATE CARE

From the patient perspective, salient questions remain: What do patients want in terms of compassionate care? Are these expectations being met? In the emancipatory theory of compassion in nursing, Georges (2013) outlines how compassion frees an individual from suffering and is situated when the "unspeakable" (p. 6) is addressed. For Georges (2011, 2013), the unspeakable blocks compassion, is powerful, and has the potential to create violence against patients. She uses an extreme example from Nazi Germany and the treatment of prisoners as they became objects, the subject of what was not spoken. They were prisoners looked upon as unfeeling things (never overtly stated); therefore, their treatment was rationalized and sanctioned. Georges views the emancipatory theory of compassion as an acknowledgment of power that is central to praxis and describes how both nurses and patients may suffer. Georges (2013) sees opportunities in educating nurses to view compassion more broadly, within a paradigm of power and bias.

In a study from the United Kingdom by Bramley and Matiti (2014), 10 patients in a large teaching hospital, via in-depth, semi-structured interviews, reported three overarching themes:

> (1) What is compassion: knowing me and giving me your time, (2) understanding the impact of compassion: how it feels in my shoes and (3) being more compassionate: communication and the essence of nursing. (p. 2790)

Congruent with Georges' theory (2013), when patients become objects, room numbers, or diagnoses/surgical procedures, we lose sight of their humanity. In contrast, the relational aspect of care—that is, patient-centered care—allows us as nurses to acknowledge suffering and the experiences of the patient. Giving our time is an indicator of compassion; it is a resource that, when lacking, interferes with delivering compassionate care. The culture of the unit was also seen as a barrier when it served to dehumanize the patient—and when it dehumanized the nurses (Bramley & Matiti, 2014). Again, we see how compassion may serve as both prevention and antidote to those who have experienced trauma—especially our patients.

TRAUMA-INFORMED REFLECTION

If we assume compassion is a virtue that one consciously chooses to show others, recall a time when someone you encountered needed to be shown compassion. How did you respond? Was this in a personal or a professional context? Did you show compassion differently, depending upon the social role you were occupying at the time (sister/brother, girlfriend/boyfriend, nursing student/professional nurse)? How do you feel after showing compassion? Drained? Energized? Both?

WAYS OF KNOWING THROUGH A TRAUMA-INFORMED LENS

How do we, on our journey to becoming nurses and new practitioners in the profession, "know" how to render care and comfort to patients and peers? Moreover, how do we offer comfort in a trauma-informed manner? One of the most challenging aspects of nursing is defining what we do in a way that is comprehensive and comprehensible. Why? Because we do such a varied number of mental and physical tasks and have such a rich spectrum of responsibilities within our professional conduct. Unlike several other healthcare professionals, educationally, we range from associate degreed nurses to advanced practice and doctoral-prepared individuals. Translating the essence of nursing needs to be both conceptual and useful in pragmatic communications with others.

One of the most powerful approaches to organizing nursing's approach to patient care is "ways of knowing" (Carper, 1978; Chinn & Kramer, 2015). These ways of knowing also reflect what we value in nursing practice, or what is important to us. The four original ways of knowing developed by Carper (1978):

> The four patterns are distinguished according to logical type of meaning and designated as: (1) empirics, the science of nursing; (2) esthetics, the art of nursing; (3) the component of a personal knowledge in nursing; and (4) ethics, the component of moral knowledge in nursing. (p. 14)

A fifth type of knowing was introduced by Chinn and Kramer (2015) and is especially relevant in today's society: emancipatory knowing. This knowledge is "the human capacity to be aware of and critically reflect on the social, cultural, and political status quo and to determine how and why it came to be that way" (Chinn & Kramer, 2015, p. 5). To fully demonstrate this type of knowing, the other four ways must be integrated into the nurse's practice. Emancipatory knowledge allows the nurse to broaden the conceptual landscape to include areas of social justice, hegemony, and distribution of power.

Stigmas and secrecy surrounding some traumas are being eroded. The #MeToo (n.d.) movement, established in 2006 for young women of color from disadvantaged backgrounds, gained prominence in 2017 and 2018 as more women come forward who are survivors of sexual violence. Another organization that has caught significant media attention is the Times Up movement, established in 2018 by women in Hollywood who are pushing back against sexual harassment and assault as well as unequal payment practices that appear to have a long cultural history of acceptance due to the loci of power. Treatment of immigrants into the US is also evidence of emancipatory knowing and is especially relevant to nurses providing care.

Nurses are socialized in school to think locally, not hegemonically/economically/politically: Their organization of employment becomes their world. They are physically located in this environment, typically, for 12-hour shifts. They return home, often spent physically and emotionally. While we have concerns of a broader context that impacts point-of-service, our energy conservation often dictates that these concerns are best addressed by others.

Nurses can no longer afford to stay on the periphery of these conversations, however. Our interests are served by inclusion in conversations, actions that push us beyond our comfort zones.

The Nurses on Board Coalition (2018) formed in 2014 with the goal of having 10,000 nurses on boards of directors by 2020. The website allows for all interested nurses to place their names ("I want to serve") for notification of board opportunities across the nation. We have heard well-founded critiques of organizational environments from nurses. To ensure this feedback is heard and information to build stronger, fairer, sustainable organizations is forwarded, nurses need to be involved.

APPLICATION OF WAYS OF KNOWING: CASE STUDY

Think about this scenario. A newly licensed community health nurse, Jenna, makes a home visit to an older adult, Claire, recently discharged from the hospital with orders for wound care of a leg ulcer secondary to uncontrolled type 2 diabetes. The patient is also a grandmother who has taken in her two young grandchildren, ages 3 and 4 years. The older child, Brittany, has been demonstrating inappropriate sexual behaviors (such as pulling at others' clothing, excessive masturbation, and going up to adults and rubbing her genitals against them). In Jenna's presence, the grandmother scolds and punishes the child, feeling embarrassed and uncertain about how to deal with this behavior. Claire also reports that Brittany will often overeat and feels sick after dinner. She has been hoarding food in her room, which draws insects. Jenna listens intently and is approached by the child, who seems overly active and somewhat aggressive with the younger sibling. More specific data is collected (history of neglect), but there are major gaps in what Brittany experienced while in the care of her birthparents, both of whom experienced substance use issues and dependency on opioids. How does this nurse apply her ways of knowing?

EMPIRICAL KNOWLEDGE

When we gather information from the medical record, when laboratory values are reviewed, when a heart sound is assessed, and when we intervene based on information collected through our senses, we have used empirical knowledge. This type of knowledge is highly valued in healthcare. Researchers and educators also tend to emphasize the knowledge that we gather through our senses. Such knowledge is considered objective and can be verified with others because it represents "facts." The assumption of such knowledge is that there is an objective reality that can be assessed and tested with deductive reasoning and that ultimately provides us with universal laws. One assumes a truth through the application of such laws. Chemistry, biology, physics, and other natural or pure sciences offer the best examples of such objective laws.

Evidence of such knowledge is also in the prescribing of medicines, of finding telomeres and genetic codes, and in the orders received from physicians. Nurses must have empirical knowledge to practice safely and effectively. Understanding pharmacology, pathophysiology, anatomy and physiology, and the evidence that supports nursing interventions makes us competent nurses. But be aware that singular application of science in our practice, while highly valued, is limited when in isolation.

Utilizing empirical knowledge of trauma supports competent care. Our application of this information may avoid misinterpretations of perceptions and behaviors that arise from traumatic experiences. In the case of Claire, Jenna considers anatomy and physiology of the skin and underlying tissue and the physical trauma of the ulcer to the body. She also considers the effect of the disease state and discusses Claire's diet intake, with an emphasis on carbohydrates and protein. Jenna is careful to document her assessment of the wound and follow the wound care orders to appropriately ensure optimal healing. Last, Jenna discusses appropriate hygiene with Claire and instructs Claire on clean dressing changes. She ensures that Claire has adequate supplies to ensure dressing changes are performed as ordered. Claire seems to understand and is able to repeat the procedure to Jenna, but she is preoccupied with Brittany's behaviors.

ESTHETICS/THE ART OF NURSING

We believe the optimal nursing care has a strong component of esthetic knowledge. The nurse who crafts care as an art understands that there are phenomena associated with care that may be unspoken, assessed indirectly. The reason behind patients' actions becomes important, and the nurse is a transformative individual in not merely assessing what can be empirically measured but also what is felt through insight and empathy (Carper, 1978) and, with this knowledge, the nurse extends comfort (Morse, 2018). When a nurse delivers care with esthetic knowledge, the patient becomes a person, not an object. Barriers are broken, and meaning is captured while interactions and connections take place (Chinn & Kramer, 2015). There is a balance, a rhythm, a duality in which barriers are absent (Carper, 1978).

We believe that the art of nursing is at a critical juncture. Pressure within the organization and the current structures of healthcare delivery can negatively affect the art of nursing. Time is needed to create connections, to listen, to understand meaning, and to provide care with a transcendent beauty. Some would argue that this way of knowing comes with time spent as a nurse, with experiences we learn from. This is linked with personal knowing, which we discuss in the next section.

In our case study, we return to Jenna, Claire, and Brittany. Jenna has done an excellent job of delivering care based on empirical knowledge. She has focused on the presenting problem: a disease process that has caused a leg ulcer, with susceptibility to infection. Jenna's teaching has been appropriate for Claire (educational level/health literacy), and Jenna has ensured that Claire understands the instructions by having her repeat them. So, what is missing?

Jenna also uses esthetic knowing as the visit ensues. She notes that Brittany's externalizing behaviors are of concern, and Claire has described further behaviors and her inability to understand them. Gaps remain in the history, however, and Jenna cannot verify whether there has been past sexual abuse but knows this is a possibility. Jenna sits across from Claire and discusses how children may act out sexually and when this is a sign of stress, neglect, or something more. She guides her in what to say, nonpunitively, so that Brittany can be redirected without shame. She encourages Claire, who has been avoiding Brittany, to connect with her in ways that they both are comfortable with (such as in the car, going to school, or after preschool). She advises her to observe Brittany's behaviors and keep a log of times when the acting out occurs, such as bath time or bedtime.

Jenna also speaks to how neglect may have affected Brittany and how common food hoarding is with individuals who have experienced food insecurity and felt hunger. She uses intuition to help Claire destigmatize Brittany's behaviors by creating a new reality for Claire to consider. Jenna offers suggestions about how to give Brittany control over having a snack to take to her room—something that is negotiated between the two of them. A plastic bag could be used to avoid attracting insects. Jenna discusses how to counsel Brittany when she overeats, emphasizing there is food available if she is hungry after the meal. Jenna and Claire talk about safety and how Brittany and Claire both need to feel safe in their environment. She also wants to view the family as a whole and knows that Claire may be experiencing secondary trauma with increasing levels of stress. Jenna's empirical knowledge also points to the relationship between wound healing and stress; by sensing both what is verbalized and that which is encompassed in the totality of the patient experience, Jenna practices the art of nursing in a trauma-informed way.

PERSONAL KNOWING

Nursing brings a mirror close to our faces in ways not found in other professions. Because we interface with other individuals in states of crisis and extreme vulnerability, we cannot afford to be less than self-aware. In personal knowing, the goal is to "know the self" (Carper, 1978, p. 18). This knowledge invites a dialogue with others characterized by authenticity and a feeling of being centered. The nurse is able to use the Self as a vehicle of humanness and meeting the patient in a similar fashion. In personal knowing, you accept ambiguity and uncertainty and suspend premature conclusions (Carper, 1978). Our attitudes, opinions, mind-sets, biases, and awareness of how others see us contribute to our knowledge of the Self. Chinn and Kramer (2015) discuss dimensions of this type of knowing: spiritual, the Self in relation to others (for example by giving, empowerment, the value of human life, and community), discovery of Self, and "unknowing" (pp. 115–117). Nurses witness the entry to and departures from earthly lives. We are witnesses to miracles and selfless acts, and in making sense of these, a spiritual component is developed that contributes to our sense of Self. In giving care to others, we learn of ourselves.

Jenna knows the Self in a deliberate and conscious way (Chinn & Kramer, 2015); she is comfortable listening to what Claire describes and seeks to connect with her through therapeutic listening techniques. Based on her experience, she renders care in a way she knows is safe and effective. Her reactions to Brittany's behaviors are analyzed internally, and she examines her biases and assumptions. In this way, she continues to discover the Self as an ongoing process. She seeks further knowledge in areas she assesses as lacking, such as what is appropriate developmental sexual behavior and what should be concerning. By "unknowing" (Chinn & Kramer, 2015, p. 117), she leaves a cognitive mind-set of being open to new information that she was unaware of.

ETHICAL KNOWING

The complexity of ethical knowing is often contextualized within uncertainty and ambiguity. This type of knowing is based on what is morally right and wrong (Carper, 1978). The American Nurses Association (ANA) Code of Ethics for Nurses with Interpretive Statements (2015) offers nine provisional statements as guidance into the ethical responsibilities as professionals. Translating these provisional statements (ANA, 2015) with a trauma focus includes:

- Practicing with respect and compassion should include providing for safety and fostering trust.

- Our commitment to the patient, family, group, or community means accurate interpretation of behaviors and needs that traumatic events may have created.

- Advocating and protecting our patients includes creating an environment that minimizes traumatization and retraumatization by recognizing services most likely to have these outcomes.

- Taking responsibility and being accountable for the care offered creates a charge for us as professionals to be trauma-educated.

- Nurses' commitment to self-care speaks to compassion fatigue and secondary trauma.

- Supporting an ethical work environment incorporates psychological safety for the nurse, coworkers, and patients.

- Advancing the profession spans educating others in how to avoid patient trauma and retraumatization in healthcare settings.

- Collaborations with others include mental health professionals and referrals to treatment that may be outside the typical scope of case management.

- Communicating nursing values through our professional organizations spans the tenet of preventing, mitigating, and treating traumatic stress.

Jenna suspects that Brittany has experienced past sexual abuse and knows Claire's resources are being depleted. She learns that Claire has delayed applying for foster parent status because the forms are overwhelming and tedious. By being a foster parent, however, Jenna knows that Claire will have access to resources that would help both her and her two granddaughters. Jenna contacts the county Department of Child Services (DCS) office and requests services to aid Claire in finishing the paperwork and accessing services as a relative caregiver. She speaks to the case manager about Brittany's behaviors, emphasizing that she believes the child should be evaluated, and visits to the birthparent's home should be assessed for safety and supervised. Jenna documents carefully so that other professionals can access this information.

EMANCIPATORY KNOWING

The importance of emancipatory knowing, added by Chinn and Kramer (2015) as the fifth way of knowing, cannot be overstated. Societal and global changes have increased the risk for trauma. The events of 9/11 altered what safety means for all Americans. Each time we fly and are processed through security, we are reminded of how unsafe the world can be. Scandals in institutions such as the Catholic Church, higher education, and political offices often bring discouragement and secondary trauma from consuming the latest national and international news reports.

Still, emancipatory knowledge is about understanding power and how it is divided, and thus, about social justice. Social determinants of health and disadvantaged individuals call to us to have a reckoning of privilege. The question posed to us when we began our careers still remains unanswered: Is healthcare a right or a privilege? A one-payer system, such as that found in Canada, may help us understand ways in which to reach more people who need healthcare services in America because it would appear our current system is not sustainable, and it does not provide healthcare to all who need it.

When applying her emancipatory knowledge, Jenna understands that relative or kinship placements have surged with the opioid crisis in the US. As birthparents have been unable to care for their children and the foster care system balloons, county service workers have sought relatives to assume children's care. Knowing that resources are often scarce and that social determinants of health impact health outcomes, Jenna's plan is to comprehensively address the needs of Claire, Brittany, and her younger sister. This means supporting the management of chronic health conditions, mental health issues, and typical development knowing that contextualized, culturally sensitive collaborations with additional service providers will be necessary. Jenna also knows that she will need to advocate for this family with the DCS, obtaining referrals with providers who accept patients with Medicare and Medicaid health coverage, and school officials. Jenna also contacts her community foundation and requests to sit on the board to advocate for nontraditional families.

In Table 6.1, we map trauma-informed knowing onto the nurses' ways of knowing (Carper, 1978; Chinn & Kramer, 2015). This organizing framework assists in accurate assessment and planning of interventions for those who have experienced stressful events.

TABLE 6.1 TRAUMA-INFORMED KNOWING

WAY OF KNOWING*	TRAUMA-INFORMED KNOWING
Empirical knowing	What literature and evidence support my interventions?
	What does the science tell me about trauma, traumatic stress, and PTSD?
	How do I recognize the physical changes within the brain and body for those experiencing and remembering trauma? Are there vital sign/cardiovascular changes, hypervigilance, and other outward signs of PTSD?
Esthetic/The art of nursing	How do I achieve a rhythm with my patient—a mutual, balanced interaction in which I bring a sense of safety and trust?
	How do I best allow the person to share his narrative with me at his own pace?
	How do I communicate that we are establishing something sacred between us that I will honor and protect?
	How do I convey empathy, caring, and comfort that focuses on safety, negotiating control, and an openness to learning?
Personal knowing	How do I enrich my care and comfort with my own knowledge of Self?
	How do I avoid a premature closing of information based on my own personal biases, assumptions, and experiences?
	How can I best inventory my own mind-set and behaviors related to this individual's trauma? How do I react to the "unspeakable"?
	What is difficult for me to hear and explore? Why is this difficult?
Ethical knowing	How do I create an ethical plan with the individual who has experienced trauma, weighing safety, trust, and what is right?
	How do I clarify the best course of action in collaboration with other professionals and the individual?
	How do I make sense of injuries inflicted by others and hear the narratives of those traumatic experiences without depleting my own resources?

continues

TABLE 6.1 TRAUMA-INFORMED KNOWING (CONT.)

WAY OF KNOWING*	TRAUMA-INFORMED KNOWING
Emancipatory knowing	How do I recognize political and policy changes that are needed to decrease trauma, violence, and injuries?
	How do I mobilize resources to impact changes to protect those most vulnerable to trauma and traumatic events?
	How do I become empowered as an individual change agent to support those who have been impacted by past trauma?

Sources: Carper, 1978; Chinn & Kramer, 2015

TRAUMA-INFORMED REFLECTION

Think about a time when you were with a friend, family member, or patient who had experienced trauma. How did you apply the ways of knowing when you interacted with the person? Looking at the five ways of knowing, which ones did you apply the most often? Which ways of knowing did you use the least? Moving forward, how would you change your discourse based on this information?

WAYS OF KNOWING: KEY POINTS

Taken together, the five ways of knowing (Carper, 1978; Chinn & Kramer, 2015) are powerful conceptualizations of what we do and what we know. We also believe that these powerful mechanisms craft trauma-informed conversations and interventions with individuals under our care. As those who created this framework knew (Carper, 1978; Chinn & Kramer, 2015), a balance between these dimensions is critically important. Using one way of knowing in isolation can significantly impact the quality of care offered. For example, if a nurse focuses on empirical knowledge, she won't be able to see the different needs the patient brings to her. The caregiver may come across as task oriented, lacking warmth and empathy, and even objectifying the patient. You can readily understand that this may retraumatize individuals who may be struggling with posttraumatic issues of safety and trust.

Similarly, if knowledge of Self is emphasized, competency in care may be weakened (lacking the science behind the interventions). This caregiver, while open to understanding more and growing as an individual, may miss important cues about brain and body functioning post trauma. Emancipatory knowledge may be closed off because of the concentration on Self. The individual who presents to a nurse focused on Self may endure someone too quick to draw conclusions based on personal experiences. Again, retraumatization may result.

A nurse who is fixated on ethical principles may overlook the risks to safety of the traumatized individual. For example, an undocumented immigrant may avoid seeking healthcare services due to fear of being deported. The nurse, in contrast, may ethically feel obligated to obtain services for this individual. The ethical principles of benevolence and distributive justice may be violated. If the nurse overemphasizes these principles, she jeopardizes the ability to offer any services to the individual, who has much to risk.

Therefore, to engage an individual in a trauma-informed, therapeutic way, our approach should be one of balance. Although the five ways of knowing help us understand our practice approach, nursing theory also enlightens us as we organize interventions around concepts and relational statements. Three nursing theories are highlighted in the next section.

THEORY TO THE RESCUE

As a practice-dominated profession, nurses tend to be unaware of the relationship between theory, research, and practice. Yet to fully function as a provider, you need to appreciate the integration of all three. Theories are meant to provide sense-making (there are even common sense theories), guidance, clarity, and patterns to our work. Theories themselves can be divided into grand theories, those that comprehensively encompass nursing care, and midrange theories, those that are more adaptable to practice and clinical contexts. In this section, we describe three nurse theorists whose work provides visual acuity to our trauma-informed lens, allowing us to see organizing frameworks for the possible effects of trauma on those under our care: Hildegard E. Peplau (1909–1999), Madeleine M. Leininger (1925–2012), and Jean Watson (1940–present).

The brief review of three nursing theories serves to introduce you to their potential in organizing your TIC. Too often, people discount the value of theory in nursing. We are such a practice-driven profession that pausing to reflect what it is we do and what it is we are, we often forget about the history and current development of nursing and health-related theories. Additional nurse theorists may speak to you as you move forward in your nursing practice in a trauma-informed manner. We encourage you to reconsider the role theory may play in your nursing career.

THEORY OF INTERPERSONAL RELATIONS: HILDEGARD PEPLAU

Student nurses in prelicensure programs as well as those who specialize in psychiatric-mental health nursing will probably know Peplau's theory of interpersonal relations. Her seminal work first published in 1952, *Interpersonal Relations in Nursing: A Conceptual Frame of Reference for Psychodynamic Nursing*, set forth her beliefs about the nurse-patient relationship. She mentions "psychic trauma" intermittently throughout her work (Peplau, 1952/1991); however, it is not a primary concept. Instead, Peplau (1952/1991) lists four psychobiological experiences that influence personalities: needs, frustration, conflict, and anxiety (p. 71). Individuals reorganize and energize based on these internal experiences. Another aspect to her theory is participant observation, during which the nurse observes not only herself and the patient but also the relations between these actors (Peplau, 1997, p. 162). Peplau's writings are prophetic; she describes shifts in healthcare, technology, and social determinants, which make nurse-patient connections essential: "The new high-technology information age is already in evidence in healthcare systems" (Peplau, 1997, p. 163). Peplau (1997) refers to virtual reality replacing reality; one thinks of care delivery via telemedicine and the attention paid to electronic health records.

Further, Peplau's theory is about the three overlapping phases that characterize the evolution of the nurse-patient dyad's relationship, a relationship that to Peplau is different from other social relationships (Peplau, 1997):

- The first phase, orientation, occurs. It is a time to collect important patient information and set the tone for the relationship. It is not the time to share the nurse's personal information. During this phase, the two parties have preconceptions of one another. The nurse should be aware of these—perhaps the patient reminds the nurse of her father; perhaps the patient sees his parent in the nurse.

- The second phase, working, is when most of the building of the relationship occurs. In the psychiatric setting, social conversation is replaced with disclosures of problem areas. Peplau emphasizes four roles of the nurse: physical care, health teaching, interviewing, and counseling.

- The last phase, termination, is typically characterized by a short time frame (for example, perhaps admission to discharge/death). Peplau asserts that, "In all cases the dissolution of the relationship requires some reflection by the nurse" (p. 165).

To map our trauma paradigm onto Peplau's work, we argue that the sacredness of the nurse-patient relationship and the necessity of this relationship to feel connected to others are certainly part of TIC. The anxiety identified by Peplau (1952/1991) may be a proxy for trauma in that there are both positive and negative outcomes. In essence, Peplau's theory stands out in the trauma context because of 1) her deliberate emphasis on the nurse-patient connection, 2) the essential need for this relationship, and 3) the nurse being reflective to the dynamics and nature of the patient-nurse relationship. We care for those who have a history of trauma and need to understand the dynamics of our relationship with them.

THEORY OF CULTURE CARE DIVERSITY AND UNIVERSALITY: MADELEINE M. LEININGER

Up to this point, we've only briefly mentioned the role of culture in understanding the Event, Experience, and Effects of trauma (the three E's of trauma from Chapter 3). But it is a critical point. John serves many undergraduate and graduate students who have experienced significant trauma. On one hand, there are universal reactions to traumas that affect us; on the other hand, the interpretations of trauma (the three E's; SAM-HSA, 2014) are influenced by our cultural norms, mores, and values. John finds that establishing a sacred, safe environment is critical because he allows the individual to disclose at her own pace, giving her psychological protection. At times, for a woman born in a developing country, disclosing intimate violence is extremely difficult and frightening. Amplifying this reticence is the tragic fact that these individuals have often been victims of racial violence, which compounds feelings of fear, isolation, and disconnection from others. Slowly, but frequently, they come to trust John and begin their healing.

One pioneer in the nursing world to offer a theoretical orientation to cultural care in nursing is Madeleine Leininger, who devised the theory of culture care diversity and universality. The influence of her doctoral degree in anthropology is evident in her work. This theory was conceptualized in the 1950s and became more widely used in the 1960s (Leininger, 2007); Leininger herself sees this theory as distinct from other "mainstream nurse theorists" (Leininger, 1988, p. 154). However, the theory began to be integrated into nursing practice as culturally congruent care was accepted as critical to our professional practice (Leininger, 2007). *Emic* knowledge is held by "cultural informants as they know and practice care with their values and beliefs in their unique cultural context" (Leininger, 2007, p. 10). *Etic* knowledge, in contrast, is "outsider views of non-local or non-indigenous care values and beliefs such as those of professional nurses" (Leininger, 2007, p. 10). Comparing these two forms of knowledge—emic and etic—supports culturally congruent care.

The acceptance of qualitative forms of research, such as phenomenology, also led to acceptance of this theory. Leininger (1988) suggests that the nurse researcher presents with an etic view; therefore, she may not allow for the values held by those in the study to be accounted for (Leininger, 1988). Leininger's work stresses that nursing theories may be more appropriate to certain cultures than others, and nursing research findings may be more applicable to certain cultures than others (Leininger, 1992). Her diagrammatic representation of her theory is the Sunrise Enabler (originally, Sunrise Model), which has been refined over time (Leininger, 1988; Leininger & McFarland, 2006). The diagram, presenting the rising sun, contains major concepts of her theory, beginning with a worldview and cultural and social structure dimensions; at the bottom, transcultural care and decisions are offered and made (Leininger & McFarland, 2006). As with Peplau, Leininger (1988) was prophetic in the increasing importance of her theory, predicting that personalized care would become economically valued as part of quality healthcare services. Leading efforts, Leininger founded the Transcultural Nursing Society (2018) in the mid-1970s; today, this organization publishes a peer-reviewed journal and sponsors conferences related to transcultural education and scholarship.

Several components of Leininger's theory of culture care diversity and universality translate to optimum TIC. Her concept of cultural care universality is defined as "common, similar, or uniform meanings, patterns, values, or symbols of care that are culturally derived by humans for their well-being or to improve a human condition" (Leininger, 1988, p. 156). In other words, these are our universal truths and humanity. When a minority group is objectified and individuality is lost, there is temptation to resist common human experiences. Yet, why would traumatic events lack this human truth, regardless of race, ethnic group, or culture? Grief, loss, mourning, fear, and distrust represent our humanness as we process trauma. For example, forced separation from a competent, caring parent and the parent's child knows no cultural bounds and evokes significant, horrific trauma.

For Leininger (1988), another dimension must be accounted for: cultural care diversity. She defines that as "patterns, value, or symbols of care that are culturally derived by humans for their well-being or to improve a human condition" (p. 156). When we apply TIC, we take these culturally construed meanings and create person-centered nursing diagnoses, planning, implementation, and evaluation. Balancing our universal humanness with cultural congruent care, our TIC will be compassionate and effective.

THEORY OF TRANSPERSONAL CARING/CARING SCIENCE: JEAN WATSON

In 2016, when Karen was inducted into the American Academy of Nursing, she had the honor of meeting Jean Watson. Karen had never met this renowned nursing theorist, and when introduced at Watson's table and asked to join the group, she worried she was imposing. But the person who greeted Karen was a warm, open, friendly woman who put her arm around her and happily posed for a picture to commemorate the evening. There was such a relaxed demeanor to Watson, characteristic of one who knows the Self and understands the world. She was humble, approachable, and welcoming. This memory remains vivid in Karen's mind, remarkable for such a brief interaction and testimony to the person Watson is.

Author or coauthor of more than 30 books, with recently published works by other authors surrounding her theory and approach to caring science, Watson's influence in nursing has been profound (Watson, 2018). With graduate degrees in mental health nursing and educational counseling and psychology, her work translates easily to the trauma context. Located in Boulder, Colorado, the Watson Caring Science Institute (Watson, 2018) offers coaching programs, graduate education opportunities, and conference information.

Many times, nursing has been referred to as a caring science with the concept of caring at the nexus of our profession. And while other theories place caring as the primary concept, Watson's work continues to be integrated into the realms of education, practice, and research. There is a complexity to this theory that reflects the complexities of nursing. Attention is paid to the nurse and practicing with lovingkindness toward self and patients; compassion is frequently discussed (Siztman & Watson, 2018). In a taped interview with Watson, conducted by Fawcett (2002), Watson described her theory:

> The theory is about a different way of being human, a different way of being present, attentive, conscious, and intentional as the nurse works with another person. (p. 215)

More specifically, Watson posits Ten Caritas Processes (Watson, 2008). *Caritas* is a dominant value in her theory, meaning an "integration of love and care that reminds us of the sacred work of healthcare" (Horton-Deutsch & Anderson, 2018, p. 6). These processes describe lovingkindness, authenticity, being sensitive, sustaining relationships, problem-solving, creating a healing environment, and allowing for miracles (Watson, 2008). Such sacred acts are about the nurse being mindful and present and serve as a contrast to the dominant medical paradigm of logical positivism and empirical knowledge.

This overview simplifies the enormity and depth of Watson's theory, and we encourage you to explore it more closely. In translating this work onto our TIC, there are multiple and obvious connections. First, the duality of transpersonal relationships allows us, as we enter into the trauma context, to identify that which may cause trauma for ourselves as we create sacred acts and relationships with our patients. Being mindful, compassionate, and present facilitates the patient into feeling safe, connecting with us, and learning to trust again. An authentic nurse will help the patient mourn, while allowing us to understand what is within our scope to change. Perhaps most of all, Watson's theory calls to demonstrate lovingkindness to ourselves and those who have been traumatized.

PROGRAMS FOR SUPPORTING MENTAL HEALTH POST TRAUMA

As we wind the chapter to a close, we turn to community-based programs aimed to address mental health in larger groups. With an urgent need to address mental health needs throughout our communities, as well as disaster relief efforts that include lay individuals, programs have thrived that provide such training. Here we take a closer look at two programs that apply the tenets of trauma-informed practices: Mental Health First Aid and Psychological First Aid.

MENTAL HEALTH FIRST AID

For myriad reasons, the need for behavioral/mental health services exceeds professional behavioral/mental health resources. In response to supporting early identification of such needs and assisting in locating resources, Mental Health First Aid, which is managed, operated, and disseminated by the National Council for Behavioral Health (NCBH, 2018) and Missouri Department of Mental Health, became available in 2008. Hadlaczky, Hökby, Mkrtchian, Carli, and Wasserman (2014) performed a meta-analysis to examine the effectiveness of Mental Health First Aid. Three outcome measures were identified: change in knowledge, attitudes, and helping behaviors. Favorable results were revealed: a positive change in knowledge, a decrease in negative attitudes, and an increase in supportive behaviors toward those with mental health issues (Hadlaczky et al., 2014).

With an emphasis on recovery and resiliency, Mental Health First Aid covers topics such as depression and mood disorders, anxiety disorders, trauma, psychosis, and substance use disorders (NCBH, 2018). Two courses are offered: one focused on adult mental health and one on children and adolescents (12–18 years); each is approximately eight hours in length. Although there is a monetary charge, course locations may be found at https://www.mentalhealthfirstaid.org/take-a-course/.

PSYCHOLOGICAL FIRST AID

For many, the thought of an emergent situation, disaster, or terrorist attack may seem to only affect others. Yet we recall vividly how a shooting on our campus in 2014 instilled a new awareness of unpredictable and traumatic events. Karen recalls suddenly shouting, "Shelter in place!" and faculty and students running to the lower-level designated area. Karen, with about 15 colleagues, took shelter in a dark room where they used phones and computers to try to learn what was happening on campus. Unsubstantiated reports of snipers, multiple gunmen, undercover police, and multiple deaths were shared—none of which turned out to be accurate. National television fed them more information, again most of which was communicated without verification. Karen thought she heard footsteps—a clear threat to her safety because the magnitude of the shooting was simply unavailable. Finally, the group received the "All clear" message and went back to their offices.

The need to debrief and share was overwhelming. The group wanted to learn more, make sense out of what had happened: A single shooter, a student, had killed another. Karen held class two hours after the university had declared that it was once again safe to walk the campus grounds. However, many parents refused to allow their children to attend class until more was known. As a way of beginning class, Karen placed the media feed onto the projection screen, and, as a whole, the class watched the university's president calmly describe what was known. She decided that no penalties would be in place for those who had elected to miss class. She led a discussion about what the students were feeling and assessed that many of them were still confused and disoriented. Finally, she dismissed class early, offering to continue to speak to students after dismissal. The counseling center was also available to any student after the event.

We learned much that day. The need to debrief and try to make sense of such events consumed us in real time and later, after the event had ended. We wanted to feel safe. We wanted to learn the facts so that we could feel safe. Last, we learned that leadership in such instances is critical. The university president's presence and steadiness reassured us as we watched the media feed, and he answered questions with calmness and thoughtfulness. As the leader of this group of students, Karen also felt an obligation to provide a sense that it was all right; they were safe, and to promote that sense of safety, protocols (attendance) could and should be broken. Although this was a localized emergent situation, more widespread disasters are part of our life, and understanding the trauma evoked from them is important.

Based on national data, experiencing a natural disaster is the second most common type of trauma (Kessler et al., 1999). Increasing conversations about global and domestic disasters—man-made and organically driven—have spurred the development of Psychological First Aid (Brymer et al., 2006) to mitigate the immediate effects of disasters and terrorism faced by children, adolescents, adults, and families. First responders and other disaster workers may also benefit from Psychological First Aid training. The program is designed to reduce the impact of the trauma through interventions from mental health professionals and first responders via evidence-based strategies. Interventions for children and families, adults, and caretakers—those who have experienced a disaster or terror event— may be delivered in many settings, some generated by the disaster: in the field, shelters, triage areas, acute care hospitals, and temporary medical units (Brymer et al., 2006). Figure 6.1 presents survivors' positive and negative immediate reactions when faced with a disaster (Brymer et al., 2006).

◼ When Terrible Things Happen - What You May Experience

Immediate Reactions

There are a wide variety of positive and negative reactions that survivors can experience during and immediately after a disaster. These include:

Domain	Negative Responses	Positive Responses
Cognitive	Confusion, disorientation, worry, intrusive thoughts and images, self-blame	Determination and resolve, sharper perception, courage, optimism, faith
Emotional	Shock, sorrow, grief, sadness, fear, anger, numb, irritability, guilt and shame	Feeling involved, challenged, mobilized
Social	Extreme withdrawal, interpersonal conflict	Social connectedness, altruistic helping behaviors
Physiological	Fatigue, headache, muscle tension, stomachache, increased heart rate, exaggerated startle response, difficulties sleeping	Alertness, readiness to respond, increased energy

FIGURE 6.1   Psychological First Aid: When terrible things happen.
Source: Brymer et al. (National Child Traumatic Stress Network and National Center for PTSD), 2006. Reprinted with permission.

For nurses to be trauma-informed, the concept of the anniversary of the event should be considered. When doing research with adoptive families, Karen learned how some children, as the date of placement or removal from a birth family drew near, would become sad or act out. This would often confuse parents—it was a joyous day for them—until they understood that the day signified loss or trauma for the children. An anniversary of the disaster event is one example of a trigger that can cause the same level of distress as the original trauma and may lead to retraumatization

(SAMHSA, 2017). Those more at risk for retraumatization are individuals with a history of high-frequency life traumas, being disconnected socially, living and working in places that are unsafe (such as combat zones), having maladaptive coping strategies, and lack of resources and mental health services (SAMHSA, 2017). Nurses should be aware of patients' histories when they engage with them to understand behaviors and form proactive strategies to avoid or reduce retraumatization.

In the "When a Patient Dies" sidebar, we provide a scenario of a young man's death, the role of a trauma-informed supervisor, and the healing component to debriefing with someone who cares.

WHEN A PATIENT DIES

Silence filled the room as the mother, father, and sister looked down at the 18-year-old's still body. The physical body had been ravaged by acute lymphocytic leukemia, yet his face seemed to be relaxed, accepting, his startling blue eyes closed. The young man, Alex, had put up a ferocious fight over the past 12 months, enduring months of hospitalization, chemotherapy, stem cell transplants, and even radiation. In the end, his body couldn't fight the infection due to his compromised immune system. No one knew the source of the infection, but it had led to multisystem organ failure and eventually to Alex's passing.

As a pediatric ICU nurse of two years, Meg had cared for Alex several times over the past year. She was taken with his sense of humor, but also with his innocence and easygoing nature. She wondered if she would have shown such grace at the same age, given what he had to go through to treat his cancer. She'd grown attached to Alex, and they'd celebrated his remission when he was discharged last week. The infection had taken hold quickly and mercilessly. Her body felt heavy, but she offered her presence to the grieving family.

Meg tried to place her hand on the mother's shoulder, but it was instantly shaken off.

"It's this hospital's fault that my son is dead!" Alex's mother, Audrey, stated. "He didn't get that nasty infection at home. This bug is in this stupid hospital. I know for a fact that half those people didn't wash their hands before they touched him. He was beating the leukemia and would still be alive if you guys had done your jobs right."

Meg knew that Audrey's anger was part of her grief. Countering what she was saying wouldn't help. And Meg wondered if she was right. There had been several quality improvement projects on handwashing, and she, herself, knew the protocol was broken at times.

Audrey continued with her diatribe, her voice increasingly loud. Finally, her husband placed a hand on her forearm, and Audrey collapsed on the bed, quietly asking Meg to leave.

Outside of the room, Meg felt robotic, wondering how her other patients were doing, knowing lab draws were needed. She felt her face and knew that her wet cheeks were from tears. Just as she exited, the unit manager, Robin, saw Meg and looked at her face.

Quickly, Robin asked one of Meg's colleagues whether he could cover for Meg. "Hey, let's talk a minute," Robin said, gently steering Meg into her office. Robin had received the report and knew of Alex's death. She'd overheard some of Audrey's accusations, but as importantly, Robin knew the overwhelming anger behind them. Robin used Watson's caritas concept as she displayed lovingkindness and presence with Meg, a cherished colleague. She also used SAMHSA's principles of secondary stress for supervisors, disclosing some information about her past experiences with pediatric deaths and providing an approachable role model. And she applied the ways of knowing, especially esthetic and personal knowing, and interjected them into the conversation.

Over the next hour, Robin and Meg talked about Alex and the relationship that had formed. Robin allowed Meg to talk, to cry, to wonder whether Audrey was right about the death being the hospital's fault. When appropriate, Robin offered the reality of Alex's weakened condition and that it was impossible to determine where and how he had acquired the bacterial infection.

Robin used therapeutic communication techniques (for example, "this must be so hard," "your work was so thoughtful," "it sounds as if you made a difference in his care," "this isn't what was expected," and "it must have hurt to hear Audrey's accusations"). Mostly, Robin just listened and, through verbal and nonverbal communication, let Meg know that her sadness had been heard and acknowledged. After about an hour, Meg assured her that she could meet the family's needs and understood Audrey's anger.

After she felt Meg could finish her shift, Robin offered additional resources to Meg if she needed them (such as the employee assistance program and the chaplain's services). Robin followed up with Meg over the next few weeks to verify that Meg's grief was resolving.

CONCLUSIONS

Trauma-informed care (TIC) is part of competent care, an approach to patients in any healthcare context. A part of TIC, compassion needs to be shown to patients, ourselves, our peers, and members of the healthcare team. Through compassionate care, assumptions about nonadherence to treatment plans may be clarified by understanding past trauma. One way to apply TIC is through the ways of knowing (Carper, 1978; Chinn & Kramer, 2015), which allows the nurse to structure and organize care through empirical, esthetic, personal, ethical, and emancipatory knowing. In addition to the ways of knowing, select theories present concepts related to TIC and help organize nursing practice. Last, programs used to support mental health post trauma include Mental Health First Aid and Psychological First Aid.

- Part of competent nursing care is TIC; however, its implementation may create ethical dilemmas for the nurse when the principles of TIC contradict treatment plans.

- Compassion may translate into that which is offered to self, to patients, and to team members.

- Nursing knowledge and ways of knowing (Carper, 1978; Chinn & Kramer, 2015) are ways to organize TIC being implemented in patient care scenarios.

- Three nursing theorists—Hildegard Peplau, Madeleine Leininger, and Jean Watson—whose works are relevant to TIC provide our practice with organization and meaning.

- Trauma-informed interventions should respect the survivor's need for respect, information, connections, and hope; reflect the interplay between the trauma and the symptoms created post trauma; and integrate the social networks of the trauma survivor.

- Two programs, Mental Health First Aid and Psychological First Aid, support mental health post trauma.

REFERENCES

American Nurses Association. (2015). *Code of ethics for nurses with interpretive statements.* Silver Spring, MD: Author.

Apker, J., Propp, K. M., Zabava Ford, W. S., & Hofmeister, N. (2006). Collaboration, credibility, compassion, and coordination: Professional nurse communication skill sets in health care team interactions. *Journal of Professional Nursing, 22*(3), 180–189. doi:10.1016/j.profnurs.2006.03.002

Azeem, M. W., Aujla, A., Rammerth, M., Binsfeld, G., & Jones, R. B. (2011). Effectiveness of six core strategies based on trauma informed care in reducing seclusions and restraints at a child and adolescent psychiatric hospital. *Journal of Child and Adolescent Psychiatric Nursing, 24*, 11–15. doi:10.1111/j.1744-6171.2010.00262.x

Bramley, L., & Matiti, M. (2014). How does it really feel to be in my shoes? Patients' experiences of compassion within nursing care and their perceptions of developing compassionate nurses. *Journal of Clinical Nursing, 23*, 2790–2799. doi:10.1111/jocn.12537

Brymer, M., Jacobs, A., Layne, C., Pynoos, R., Ruzek, J., Steinberg, A., . . . Watson, P. (National Child Traumatic Stress Network and National Center for PTSD). (2006). *Psychological First Aid: Field operations guide* (2nd ed). Retrieved from https://www.nctsn.org/sites/default/files/resources//pfa_field_operations_guide.pdf

Carper, B. A. (1978). Fundamental patterns of knowing in nursing. *Advances in Nursing Science, 1*(1), 13–24.

Chinn, P., & Kramer, M. (2015). *Knowledge development in nursing: Theory and process* (9th ed.). St. Louis, MO: Mosby, Inc.

Fawcett, J. (2002). The nurse theorists: 21st-century updates—Jean Watson. *Nursing Science Quarterly, 15*(3), 214–219.

Fishbein, M. (2008). A reasoned action approach to health promotion. *Medical Decision Making, 28*(6), 834–844. doi:10.1177/0272989x08326092

Fishbein, M., & Ajzen, I. (1975). *Belief, attitude, intention and behavior: An introduction to theory and research*. Reading, MA: Addison-Wesley Publishing.

Georges, J. M. (2011). Evidence of the unspeakable: Biopower, compassion, and nursing. *Advances in Nursing Science, 34*(2), 130–135. doi:10.1097/ANS.0b013e31826cd8

Georges, J. M. (2013). An emancipatory theory of compassion in nursing. *Advances in Nursing Science, 36*(1), 2–9. doi:10.1097/ANS.0b013e31828077d2

Hadlaczky, G., Hökby, S., Mkrtchian, A., Carli, V., & Wasserman, D. (2014). Mental Health First Aid is an effective public health intervention for improving knowledge, attitudes, and behaviour: A meta-analysis. *International Review of Psychiatry, 26*(4), 467–475. doi:10.3109/09540261.2014.924910

Horton-Deutsch, S., & Anderson, J. (2018). *Caritas coaching: A journey toward transpersonal caring for informed moral action in healthcare*. Indianapolis, IN: Sigma Theta Tau International.

Isobel, S., & Delgado, C. (2018). Safe and collaborative communication skills: A step towards mental health nurses implementing trauma informed care. *Archives of Psychiatric Nursing, 32*, 291–296. doi:https://doi.org/10.1016/j.apnu.2017.11.017

Kessler, R. C., Sonnega, A., Bromet, E., Hughes, M., Nelson, C. B., & Breslau, N. N. (1999). Epidemiological risk factors for trauma and PTSD. In R. Yehuda (Ed.), *Risk factors for PTSD* (pp. 23–59). Washington, DC: American Psychiatric Press.

Leininger, M. M. (1988). Leininger's theory of nursing: Cultural care diversity and universality. *Nursing Science Quarterly, 1*(4), 152–160.

Leininger, M. (1992). Self-care ideology and cultural incongruities: Some critical issues. *Journal of Transcultural Nursing, 4*(1), 2–4. doi:https://doi-org.ezproxy.lib.purdue.edu/10.1177/104365969200400101

Leininger, M. (2007). Theoretical questions and concerns: Response from the theory of culture care diversity and universality perspective. *Nursing Science Quarterly, 20*(1), 9–15. doi:10.1177/0894318406296784

Leininger, M. M., & McFarland, M. R. (Eds.). (2006). *Culture care diversity and universality: A worldwide theory of nursing* (2nd ed.). Sudbury, MA: Jones & Bartlett.

Mason, H. D., & Nel, J. A. (2012). Compassion fatigue, burnout and compassion satisfaction: Prevalence among nursing students. *Journal of Psychology in Africa, 22*(3), 451–455. doi:https://doi.org/10.1080/14330237.2012.10820554

MeToo. (n.d.). You are not alone. Retrieved from https://metoomvmt.org/

Morse, J. M. (2018). The praxis theory of suffering. In J. B. Butts & K. L. Rich (Eds.), *Philosophies and theories for advanced nursing practice* (pp. 603–627). Burlington, MA: Jones & Bartlett Learning.

National Council for Behavioral Health. (2018). Mental Health First Aid: Get involved and make a difference. Retrieved from https://www.mentalhealthfirstaid.org/

Nurses on Board Coalition. (2018). About: Our story. Retrieved from https://www.nursesonboardscoalition.org/about/

Peplau, H. E. (1952/1991). *Interpersonal relations in nursing: A conceptual frame of reference for psychodynamic nursing.* New York, NY: Springer Publishing.

Peplau, H. E. (1997). Peplau's theory of interpersonal relations. *Nursing Science Quarterly, 10*(4), 162–167. doi:https://doi-org.ezproxy.lib.purdue.edu/10.1177/089431849701000407

Reyes, D. (2012). Self-compassion: A concept analysis. *Journal of Holistic Nursing, 30*(2), 81–89. doi:10.1177/0898010111423421

Rosenstock, I. M., Strecher, V. J., & Becker, M. H. (1988). Social learning theory and the health belief model. *Health Education and Behavior, 15*(2), 175–183.

Sacco, T. L., & Copel, L. C. (2018). Compassion satisfaction: A concept analysis in nursing. *Nursing Forum, 53*, 76–83. doi:10.1111/nuf.12213

Schantz, M. L. (2007). Compassion: A concept analysis. *Nursing Forum, 42*(2), 48–55.

Siztman, K., & Watson, J. (2018). *Caring science, mindful practice: Implementing Watson's human caring theory* (2nd ed.). New York, NY: Springer Publishing.

Stokes, Y., Jacob, J. D., Gifford, W., Squires, J., & Vandyk, A. (2017). Exploring nurses' knowledge and experiences related to trauma-informed care. *Global Qualitative Nursing Research, 4*, 1–10. doi:10.1177/2333393617734510

Substance Abuse and Mental Health Services Administration. (2014). *SAMHSA's concept of trauma and guidance for a trauma-informed approach.* HHS Publication No. SMA 14-4884. Rockville, MD: Author.

Substance Abuse and Mental Health Services Administration. (2017). *Tips for survivors of a disaster or other traumatic event: Coping with retraumatization.* HHS Publication No. SMA 17-5047.

Substance Abuse and Mental Health Services Administration. (2018). *Trauma-specific interventions.* Retrieved from https://www.samhsa.gov/nctic/trauma-interventions

Transcultural Nursing Society. (2018). About us. Retrieved from https://tcns.org/abouttcns/

Watson, J. (2008). *Nursing: The philosophy and science of caring* (Rev. ed.). Boulder, CO: University Press of Colorado.

Watson, J. (2018). Watson Caring Science Institute. Retrieved from https://www.watsoncaringscience.org/

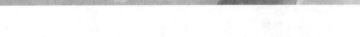

LEARNING OBJECTIVES

At the end of this chapter, you will be able to:

- Critique yourself in skills, attitudes, and knowledge in applying trauma-informed nursing care within an ethical framework.

- Argue why students on campuses are vulnerable to sexual violence; include information from NotAlone.

- Articulate the main tenets of Title IX, FERPA, and HIPAA and their implications within a trauma context.

- Be able to assess individuals' sexual orientations and gender identities along continuums.

- Recall resources and organizations that specialize in trauma information and assistance, both within and outside the nursing profession.

TRAUMA AND GEOPOLITICAL SPACES

7

PURPOSE OF THE CHAPTER

In this chapter, we juxtapose the ethical dilemmas that can result from the delivery of nursing care and those occasions when such practices contradict the foundation of trauma-informed care (TIC). We also describe privacy and the legal implications of identifying and reporting trauma (Title IX, FERPA, and HIPAA). The statement from the White House Task Force (2017) on sexual assault, with an emphasis on campus violence, is also reported. Despite trauma's prevalence in society as a whole, we focus on individuals whose gender and sexual identity may heighten their vulnerability to trauma and educate nurses on how identification can fall along continuums to optimize healthcare experiences.

ETHICS AND TRAUMA-INFORMED NURSING CARE

In Chapter 6, we discuss the five ways of knowing (Carper, 1978; Chinn & Kramer, 2015). One of the ways a nurse "knows" how to care for a patient is through ethical knowing. On a personal level, you may be aware of someone in your life who did not act in an ethical manner. Perhaps the person felt that the indiscretion was so minor it was inconsequential or created no injury to another. Maybe it was dishonesty on an examination or failure to document or report an error in clinical. Whatever the behavior or act, it fell outside ethical standards. You may also have known individuals who conduct themselves with high ethical comportment. They may not follow an easy path at times, but a path that is ethically right.

Ethical dilemmas within the context of TIC will present themselves to you as a practicing nurse. For example, what should the nurse do when a pediatric patient hospitalized on a psychiatric inpatient unit refuses her medication, but her parents insist on her taking it? This scenario becomes an ethical dilemma when the nurse is aware that the child has experienced trauma; physically forcing her to take her medication through an injection would only create more trauma (Regan, 2010). This is just one instance of how what is "right" can be in conflict with a second action that is deemed "right."

We advise nurses to uphold standards of ethical care and TIC, and prove to the world that nurses are indeed ethical professionals. For the past 16 years, nurses have been rated first in ethical and honest behavior, with military officers and grade school teachers second and third place respectively (Brenan, 2017). As psychological trauma continues to enter into our lived experiences, personal and professional conversations, and, in some instances, legacies from communities and generations, it is our ethical responsibility to be informed of the ways in which nurses can mitigate trauma's effects and promote healing.

The American Nurses Association Code of Ethics (ANA, 2015) should be embedded into our ethical way of knowing and influence our professional conduct at, as well as away from, the bedside. Understanding the deleterious effects of compassion fatigue on our ability to interact with individuals who see us as caregivers and comforters cannot be overemphasized (see Chapter 2). Similarly, screenings for depressive symptoms, anxiety, adverse childhood experiences, secondary traumatic stress symptoms, and compassion fatigue are readily available. Be aware that these are screening tools, not definitive diagnostic assessments. In other words, if you score at a high level on a scale, interpretation must be with respect to the issue of screening (you may be at risk for and be prompted for further evaluation) versus your meeting the symptom criteria for this diagnosis. There is a significant and, in our opinion, ethical distinction that must be made between risk screening and diagnosing.

SANCTUARY MODEL

Sometimes amidst all the published literature, there is an idea that seems to rise above others as something of value, something to process and consider. We came across such an idea in the thoughts of Sandra Bloom (2000, 2017; Bloom & Sreedhar, 2008), whose work began with inpatient psychiatric patients and their recovery from trauma. *Sanctuary* is described as a "place of refuge from danger, threat, injury, and fear" (Bloom & Farragher, 2011, p. 4). Bloom began broadly, helping patients overcome trauma. She also included people working in service organizations whose primary mission is to help children and families recover from trauma. With several books and a Sanctuary Institute, the model has grown to encompass organizational change and our society in a "whole culture approach" as we learn how an organization's culture affects the delivery of care (Community Works, 2018). Bloom recognizes the effects of such services on people within the organizations and uses analogies to help us understand trauma at individual and system levels (such as organizational hyperarousal, loss of emotional management, and organizational learning disabilities; Bloom & Farragher, 2011). There appears to be a paradox then, as providers attempt to provide relief from trauma to those they serve while being traumatized themselves due to an organizational culture that breeds trauma from factors such as excessive workloads, poor communication, and overwhelming demands for services (Bloom & Farragher, 2011).

S.E.L.F.: SAFETY, EMOTIONS, LOSS, AND FUTURE

Written primarily for those who provide human services related to children and families, such as social work and mental health professionals
(Bloom & Farragher, 2011), the principles of the Sanctuary Model apply
to the delivery of healthcare services in general. We also see overtures
of Chinn and Kramer's (2015) emancipatory knowledge as it applies to
the self and nurses delivering post-trauma care in healthcare organizations and experiencing compassion fatigue. One implementation tool and
framework described by Bloom (2000, 2017) and Bloom and Sreedhar
(2008) is S.E.L.F.: Safety, Emotions, Loss, and Future. These are also seen
as domains where disruptions may occur. Bloom (2000) succinctly states
how those with trauma histories are affected:

> Victims of overwhelming life experiences have difficulty stay-
> ing safe, find emotions difficult to manage, have suffered many
> losses, and have difficulty envisioning a future. As a result,
> they are frequently in danger, lose emotional control (or are so
> numb that they cannot access their emotions), have many signs
> of unresolved loss, and are stuck in time, haunted by the past
> and unable to move into a better future. (pp. 52–53)

EMOTION MANAGEMENT

Safety means physical and psychological safety, but also social and moral
safety (Bloom, 2017). Emotion management is a task we work on throughout our lives and when highly contentious issues are thrust upon us. As
adults, we need to be able to manage our reactions and expressions related
to them appropriately. Loss should be honored and anticipated when
change is considered. Ownership of who will lose as change is proposed
should also occur. Future (originally called emancipation; Bloom, 2000)
refers to what we want to achieve and what is desired through common
values, reducing resistance (Bloom, 2017). The Sanctuary Model and
S.E.L.F. are tools to improve quality services to those who are served, improve quality of life to those who serve them, and improve organizational
cultures in a trauma-informed way.

We talked in the introduction about your own trauma script and how your journey as a nurse might prompt some of these past experiences into an awareness of your thoughts and behaviors. The purpose of this discussion has been to support an analysis of trauma confronting both nurses and their patients. Now we'd like you to put this information together by synthesizing this discussion and mapping it onto you as an individual and as a (student or new) nurse. (See the "Trauma-Informed Reflection" sidebar.)

TRAUMA-INFORMED REFLECTION

Think about your life experiences and how they have shaped your world. Next, think about your present understanding of psychological trauma and how events may have affected you as an individual and as a professional nurse. After reading this book, what sense-making activities have provided growth to you? What insights have been gained? How has this new knowledge changed you? What strategies do you now possess as an individual and professional nurse that will help you prevent, mitigate, and heal from psychological trauma? Thinking of organizations, how will emancipatory knowledge and the Sanctuary Model (how culture affects care) influence you as part of a healthcare system?

TRAUMA AND SEXUAL VIOLENCE: NOTALONE

Trauma extends into different spaces of society. One of those spaces is violence against women. Indeed, we opened this book with a story of a young woman who experienced and survived a sexual assault while a student at a university. NotAlone was created in January 2014 in connection with a White House Task Force to Protect Students from Sexual Assault (White House Task Force). This task force created the following goals: to raise awareness of the frequency of sexual assault, to communicate to survivors that they are not alone and there are resources to help, to guarantee that colleges and universities develop a comprehensive plan to keep students safe, and to support schools as they implement Title IX of the Education Amendments of 1972 (White House Task Force, 2017).

A second report from the White House Task Force was issued in 2017 and was shaped by the thousands of women and men (remember, it is not only women who are sexually assaulted) who came forward to share their stories of survival post trauma. Included in this report are the findings of the Campus Climate Survey Validation Study (Krebs, Lindquist, Berzofsky, Shook-Sa, & Peterson, 2016). The findings of this survey, summarized by the White House Task Force (2017), are concerning, yet they increase awareness as to the extent of this problem (pp. 9–10):

- 1 in 5 women and 1 in 14 men experienced sexual assault while in college.

- For female bisexual and transgender students, victimization rates are even higher. More than 1 in 4 transgender students and more than 1 in 3 bisexual students experienced sexual assault while in college.

- The highest rates of sexual assault occurred during the first three months of the school year: August, September, and October. This was especially true for first-year students.

- Students rarely report rape to school authorities. Of the 2,380 students who indicated that they had experienced rape (out of the 25,000 surveyed), only 170 students—or 7%—reported the rape to school authorities.

- When students did tell someone about a sexual assault, they were much more likely to tell a roommate, friend, or family—not law enforcement or a school official.

The White House Task Force has been true to fulfilling its original goals. The Department of Justice, Office on Violence Against Women has developed guidelines for schools K–12, universities, and colleges to follow as well as resources (see Notalone.gov and www.Changingourcampus. org). These resources span a broad range of audiences, from sexual assault survivor guides to campus police who respond to reports of sexual assault. The span of violence encompasses domestic violence, dating violence, sexual assault, and stalking. In addition to resources for survivors, prevention and education are foci as well.

Specific to nurses and sexual assault is the SANE designation. The Sexual Assault Nurse Examiner (SANE) designation signifies the nurse has taken a forensic examination and is certified to care for individuals who have experienced sexual assault or abuse. (See the "SANE Certification" sidebar.) Developed in the mid-1970s, SANEs are in situations of high impact, interfacing with victims of sexual assault soon after the injury occurs.

SANE CERTIFICATION

To be certified as a Sexual Assault Nurse Examiner (SANE) in the US, a registered nurse must complete training, which includes both classroom and clinical components, and pass a certification examination. The nurse who is SANE-certified delivers comprehensive and compassionate care to those individuals who have experienced sexual assault. The International Association of Forensic Nursing (2017) administers this certification to care for both adults and adolescents (Sexual Assault Nurse Examiner-Adult/Adolescent [SANE-A]), as well as pediatric patients (Sexual Assault Nurse Examiner-Pediatric [SANE-P]). Training usually consists of approximately 40+ hours.

EDUCATION, HEALTH, TRAUMA, AND LEGAL GUIDANCE

Federal law protects our individual rights in healthcare, education, and as part of a campus community. One common theme to these federal laws is the right to privacy. In the following sections, we discuss three such laws: HIPAA, FERPA, and Title IX.

HIPAA AND PHI

The first law, the Health Insurance Portability and Accountability Act (HIPAA) of 1996, pertains to protected health information (PHI; US Department of Health and Human Services, 2013). By now, you've probably learned about this in your clinical course. To be candid, it takes vigilance to protect such information. Prior to this law, casual conversations between healthcare workers in cafeterias and elevators would describe patients, their diagnoses, and opinions about these patients. Rightfully, this is now illegal and a violation of HIPAA (as is other sharing of information, including electronic patient records and transmissions by paper or orally). The ethical component to this law is obvious. Think of the potential trauma when health information is shared inappropriately, without an individual's permission or awareness. We believe that prior to HIPAA, an individual lost certain rights when becoming a patient. Healthcare providers erroneously believed that such information no longer was under the control of the person who entered into a healthcare organization. Fortunately, HIPAA is there to safeguard our privacy, as well as our patients'.

Be aware of the consequences of sharing PHI, which include termination of employment, fines, and other sanctions. Also be aware of the need you may have to debrief after witnessing a particularly impactful clinical situation—and you will face these. You'll need to process the experience, make sense of it. Think now, proactively, about how to do this within HIPAA guidelines.

FERPA

We leave the context of healthcare and enter into federal laws that serve to protect the individual in educational settings. The Family Educational Rights and Privacy Act (FERPA; US Department of Education, 2018) protects students' educational records and applies to organizations that receive funds from the Department of Education. In summary, FERPA transfers the rights from the parents to the individual when the individual turns 18. There are instances when certain parties may access certain educational information, but restrictions hold under the law. For example, institutions have the right to disclose certain directory information, unless the student elects to opt out. For our discussion, it is important to note that faculty have a responsibility to act ethically when discussing students' performances. Posting of grades needs to be done in a manner that protects students' privacy so that other students cannot identify peers' grades. Again, if sensitive information were to be shared in a way that violated a student's rights under FERPA, a federal law would be broken.

TITLE IX

The third federal law that is pertinent to our discussion is Title IX of the Education Amendments of 1972 (Title IX):

> Title IX protects students, employees, applicants for admission and employment, and other persons from all forms of sex discrimination, including discrimination based on gender identity or failure to conform to stereotypical notions of masculinity or femininity. All students (as well as other persons) at recipient institutions are protected by Title IX—regardless of their sex, sexual orientation, gender identity, part- or full-time status, disability, race, or national origin—in all aspects of a recipient's educational programs and activities. (US Department of Education, Office of Civil Rights, 2015, p. 1)

This law seeks to protect several parties, including students, from discrimination based on sex, gender identity, and other nonconformist sexual identification within educational institutions that receive funding from the US Department of Education. This law extends beyond equity in collegiate athletics. As with HIPAA and FERPA, the subtext of this law recognizes those individuals who are in social contexts of unbalanced power (provider/patient; faculty and parents/student; organization/individual). In contrast, however, to HIPAA and FERPA, Title IX specifically addresses sexual discrimination. Organizations are charged with identifying a Title IX coordinator; launching an investigation into harassment, discrimination, and other violations; and providing training to mandatory reporters of violations (for example, administrators, staff with supervisory responsibilities, academic advisors, and resident assistants). Title IX classifies sexual harassment as including sexual violence/sexual assault, relationship violence (one type is stalking), sexual exploitation, and unwelcome sexual contact. The definition of consent is important in this law; consent is given freely and voluntarily. Consent cannot be inferred from incapacitation (lack the ability to rationally give consent) and may be withdrawn at any time. Alcohol is frequently a factor in sexual assaults. Regardless, the victim should never be blamed for an assault, and both men and women may be victims of sexual violence. However, many assaults are never reported.

TRAUMA-INFORMED SCHOOLS: K–12

Those in education are beginning to listen to the messages related to creating environments that are safe and conducive to learning. The tragedy of the Columbine High School shooting and bombing in April 1999 changed how we thought of schools being solely a place of learning. Now, the public, parents, and students view schools as potential sites of violence and trauma. The good news is that educators have made significant advances in supporting safe physical spaces. These educators have also begun to provide concrete interventions to children and adolescents. Organizations are sponsoring national conferences on "trauma-informed schools" for K–12 schools. The demand for such knowledge is impressive.

Specific to lesbian, gay, bisexual, transgender, queer, and questioning (LGBTQ) students in K–12 schools is GLSEN (pronounced glisten). This organization conducts research and advocates for LGBTQ individuals who are vulnerable to harassment and bullying (GLSEN, 2018). The values of GLSEN (2018) speak to an inclusive and diverse environment for learning, regardless of race, sexual orientation, and gender identity/expression.

TRAUMA-INFORMED REFLECTION

Is there someone in your world—a family member or friend—who has been sexually harassed or assaulted, or a victim of violence? What is the person's gender and sexual orientation? Was this a factor in the traumatic event? What are the ethical and legal implications of the violence? How did you react to this news? Knowing the trauma-informed approaches discussed in this book, how would you communicate and interact differently based on what you have learned? Knowing about secondary trauma, what processes are you now aware of to increase your resiliency?

SEXUAL ORIENTATION AND GENDER IDENTITY

In Chapter 1, we made it a point to emphasize that anyone, regardless of privilege, class, or race, can and does experience trauma. Yet the statistics from the White House Task Force (2017) demonstrate that those whose sexual orientation and gender identity differ from mainstream norms may be particularly vulnerable. We healthcare providers have an ethical responsibility to deliver not only TIC but also informed, competent care. Figure 7.1 offers continuums of biological sex, gender identity, gender expression, and sexual orientation. These spaces allow for understanding how individuals view their sexuality and gender.

In 2011, the Institute of Medicine (today known as the National Academy of Medicine) captured the heightened prevalence and unique causes of violence and trauma that LGBT individuals endure. Stigma and marginalization, difficulties across the life span, and lack of healthcare provider training were concerns raised in the IOM (2011) report. More recent resources offer such training and attempt to decrease stigma. The National LGBT Health Education Center (a program of the Fenway Institute, 2018) offers free continuing education, publications and toolkits, and consultation. There are downloadable guides for healthcare organizations, including how to collect data on sexual orientation and gender identity.

To fully understand stigma and marginalization, it is important to be aware of how these affect the health of an individual. Minority stress theory, developed by Meyer (2003), offers a framework of understanding. With a nexus or focal point of stress to the model, Meyer (2003) explores different types of chronic stress that arise from stigmatization. Within an environment, Meyer (2003) conceptualized distal minority stress processes ("prejudice events: discrimination and violence") and proximal minority stress ("expectations of rejection, concealment, and internalized homophobia"; Meyer, 2003, p. 679). Elements from other models of minority stress form the background to this model: personal predispositions, biological factors, ongoing situations, and other perceptions and ability to cope (Meyer, 2003). The outcome of this model is mental health status (positive or negative). We can see elements of the major concepts within our trauma discussion throughout this model. For instance, resiliency may be part of the personal predispositions and biological factors, or the ability to cope. The three E's (Event, Experience, and Effects; Substance Abuse and Mental Health Services Administration [SAMHSA], 2014; see Chapter 3) could be mapped to the chronic distal and proximal stresses. As with any theoretical model, Meyer (2003) presents us with an organizing framework so that we can heighten our awareness of the unique dynamics and stresses, while simultaneously approaching LGBTQ individuals with the universal need for competency and compassionate care.

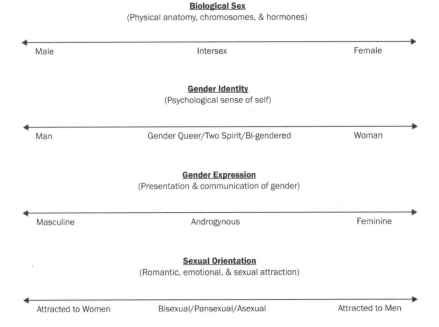

FIGURE 7.1 Continuums of sex, gender, and sexual orientation.
Source: National Child Traumatic Stress Network, Child Sexual Abuse Collaborative Group, 2014. Reprinted with permission.

RESOURCES AND ORGANIZATIONS FOR TRAUMA HELP

Trauma and TIC are becoming integrated into our daily lexicon with increasing frequency. It would be unfortunate if we were to become laissez faire with this vocabulary because, linguistically, these terms reflect more than new vocabulary: They have significance in human lives. The following are organizations that offer resources to individuals and nurses to better understand, manage symptoms of, and heal from traumatic events.

THE AMERICAN PSYCHIATRIC NURSES ASSOCIATION

The American Psychiatric Nurses Association (APNA; https://www.apna.org) is the professional nursing organization to advance the "science and education" for psychiatric-mental health (PMH) nurses (APNA, 2018). There are links to resources for understanding the impact of traumatic events, ranging from how to assist children with grief to dealing with natural disasters. More than this, the APNA provides nurses with the opportunity to network, continue education, attend conferences, share research findings, and refine caregiving. In addition, as a member, nurses can sign up for daily listserv discussions on current topics facing clinicians in delivering nursing care in behavioral healthcare settings. Based on position papers, the key points that the APNA stands for are (APNA, 2017):

- Defining the scope of psychiatric-mental health nursing

- Staffing inpatient (psychiatric) units

- Being at the forefront of violence prevention efforts

- Advocating for mental health policies that bring affordable, accessible, and integrated mental healthcare to patients

- Securing advanced practice nurses' prescriptive authority of buprenorphine for the treatment of individuals who are addicted to opiates

- Reducing and ultimately eliminating seclusion and restraint interventions for behavioral emergencies

- Implementing Screening, Brief Intervention, and Referral to Treatment (SBIRT) by PMH nurses

- Sharing of core competencies between PMH nurse practitioners and clinical nurse specialists

THE INTERNATIONAL SOCIETY OF PSYCHIATRIC-MENTAL HEALTH NURSES

The International Society of Psychiatric-Mental Health Nurses (2018; https://www.ispn-psych.org/) is a global organization that represents advanced practice nurses in mental health practice, education, and policy issues. Although trauma is not a specific focus, it is subsumed in many issues facing mental health worldwide.

SOCIETY FOR THE ADVANCEMENT OF DISASTER NURSING

The Society for the Advancement of Disaster Nursing (2018) is a collaborative site (https://disasternursing.org/) designed for any nurse to share information, education, research, policy, and practice to enhance disaster nursing preparedness. Blogs and other resources are available on the website.

THE SUBSTANCE ABUSE AND MENTAL HEALTH SERVICES ADMINISTRATION

Established in 1992, SAMHSA (https://www.samhsa.gov/) is designed to provide increased accessibility of available information related to substance use and mental health services and research in the US. In summary, SAMHSA (n.d.) "is the agency within the US Department of Health and

Human Services that leads public health efforts to advance the behavioral health of the nation. SAMHSA's mission is to reduce the impact of substance abuse and mental illness on America's communities" (para. 1). Although this mission is not specific to trauma, SAMHSA provides resources related to trauma-informed practices and caring for those affected by trauma. One of the agencies funded by SAMHSA is the National Child Traumatic Stress Network.

NATIONAL CHILD TRAUMATIC STRESS NETWORK

The National Child Traumatic Stress Network (NCTSN, n.d.; https://www.nctsn.org/) was established in 2000 as part of the Children's Health Act; its mission is to improve access, treatment, and resources to children and their families who have been impacted by trauma. This is a significant resource for healthcare providers that addresses a wide range of trauma sources. Newsletters, tools, fact sheets, and position statements address the needs of individuals, families, and communities. From military families to the effects of disasters on children, the NCTSN produces current, evidence-based literature on assessment and interventions for children exposed to trauma.

NATIONAL CENTER FOR PTSD

Although not exclusive to veterans, the National Center for PTSD has resources for both professionals and the public (US Department of Veterans Affairs, 2018; https://www.ptsd.va.gov/). Created in 1989 as a Congressional mandate, the Center offers resources and access to research, as well as vignettes of those who have been helped with TIC. With seven VA centers of excellence, the Center's mission is to improve the lives of veterans and others who have been affected by traumatic experiences. The Center also sponsors the PTSDpubs Database (see the next section).

PTSDPUBS DATABASE

The PTSDpubs Database is a freely available, searchable citation index, inclusive of all types of literature from various geographic locations, that pertains to traumatic stress (https://www.ptsd.va.gov/ptsdpubs/search_ ptsdpubs.asp). Produced by the National Center for PTSD and sponsored by the Department of Veterans Affairs, it is not limited to resources surrounding veterans (US Department of Veterans Affairs, 2017). Although it is not intended to be utilized for clinical decision-making, use of the portal is free and doesn't require login information. Retrievable information includes citations and abstracts. The years of archived literature include 1871 to the present day.

INTERNATIONAL SOCIETY FOR TRAUMATIC STRESS STUDIES

The International Society for Traumatic Stress Studies (ISTSS, n.d.; https://www.istss.org/) is "an international interdisciplinary professional organization that promotes advancement and exchange of knowledge about traumatic stress" ("ISTSS Mission"). The organization is for professionals who study traumatic stress in research studies and who treat individuals who have been affected by traumatic stress. The ISTSS presents a range of resources related to trauma, including a roster of assessment tools, policy briefs, and information related to membership. (Student membership is available.)

NATIONAL TRAUMA INSTITUTE

The National Trauma Institute (NTI, 2018; https://www.nattrauma.org/) advocates for additional federal funding and research on trauma and situates trauma as a public health problem. The NTI has a broad approach to trauma: veterans of war, older adult falls, ED visits, and injuries in general. In 2018, the NTI launched the National Trauma Research Repository, a web platform funded by the Department of Defense, for "managing research data sets to support data sharing among trauma investigators" (NTI, n.d., para. 1).

CONCLUSIONS

Geopolitical spaces occupied by those whose lives are influenced by trauma create ethical and legal considerations, as well as resources to support the rights of these individuals. Within a trauma context, unique ethical problems may surface, particularly when individuals disagree with plans of treatment and disease management. Using a Sanctuary Model (Bloom, 2000, 2017), the chronic experience of trauma can be translated by individuals, caregivers, and organizations. Federal laws, such as Title IX, FERPA, and HIPAA, protect parties from violations of privacy and stipulate guidelines in reporting sexual harassment. Marginalized groups based on sexual identity and gender identification require the nurse to understand stress theory and the potential risk factors that can arise for groups experiencing stress. As trauma is recognized to have implications outside of the home; a general movement in the US toward trauma-informed K–12 schools is rapidly growing. Resources exist to support researchers, educators, and practitioners to forward our understanding of trauma.

HIGHLIGHTS OF CHAPTER CONTENT

- Conflict between the principles of trauma-informed care (TIC) and patient care procedures embedded in organizations may create ethical and moral dilemmas.

- The Sanctuary Model (Bloom, 2000, 2017) describes how organizational cultures become traumatized through chronic stresses and create additional trauma for those working in the organization.

- NotAlone, created by the White House Task Force to Protect Students from Sexual Assault, raises awareness of sexual assault on campuses.

- The nurse who is a certified Sexual Assault Nurse Examiner (SANE) is able to competently and compassionately deliver care to victims of sexual assault.

- Three federal laws—the Health Insurance Portability and Accountability Act (HIPAA), the Family Educational Rights and Privacy Act (FERPA), and Title IX of the Education Amendments of 1972 (Title IX)—act to protect individuals' privacy and certain rights in healthcare and education.

- In the US, there is a significant movement to ensure TIC and instruction in the K–12 educational system.

- Individuals with sexual minority status are vulnerable to minority stress processes; sex, gender, and sexual orientation may be considered along continuums.

- Multiple organizations' missions are to prevent and mitigate trauma in our society. These are located both within and outside of nursing.

REFERENCES

American Nurses Association. (2015). *Code of ethics for nurses with interpretive statements.* Silver Spring, MD: Author.

American Psychiatric Nurses Association. (Spring 2017). What do we stand for? *APNA News: The Psychiatric Nursing Voice.* Falls Church, VA: Author.

American Psychiatric Nurses Association. (2018). About APNA. Retrieved from https://www.apna.org/i4a/pages/index.cfm?pageid=3334

Bloom, S. L. (2000). Creating sanctuary: Healing from systematic abuses of power. *Therapeutic Communities: The International Journal for Therapeutic and Supportive Organizations, 21*(2), 67–91.

Bloom, S. L. (2017). Some guidelines for surfing the edge of chaos, while riding dangerously close to the black hole of trauma. *Psychotherapy and Politics International.* doi:10.1002/ppi.1409

Bloom, S. L., & Farragher, B. (2011). *Destroying sanctuary: The crisis in human delivery systems.* New York, NY: Oxford University Press.

Bloom, S. L., & Sreedhar, S. Y. (2008). The Sanctuary Model of trauma-informed organizational change. *Reclaiming Children and Youth, 17*(3), 48–53.

Brenan, M. (Dec. 26, 2017). Nurses keep healthy lead as most honest, ethical profession. *Gallup.* Retrieved from https://news.gallup.com/poll/224639/nurses-keep-healthy-lead-honest-ethical-profession.aspx?g_source=CATEGORY_SOCIAL_POLICY_ISSUES&g_medium=topic&g_campaign=tile

Carper, B. A. (1978). Fundamental patterns of knowing in nursing. *Advances in Nursing Science, 1*(1), 13–24. doi:10.1097/00012272-197810000-00004

Chinn, P., & Kramer, M. (2015). *Knowledge development in nursing: Theory and process* (9th ed.). St. Louis, MO: Mosby, Inc.

Community Works. (2018). The Sanctuary Model. Retrieved from http://sanctuaryweb.com/TheSanctuaryModel.aspx

GLSEN. (2018). Improving education, creating a better world. Retrieved from https://www.glsen.org/learn/about-glsen

Institute of Medicine. (2011). *The health of lesbian, gay, bisexual, and transgender people: Building a foundation for better understanding.* Washington, DC: The National Academies Press.

International Association of Forensic Nursing. (2017). Sexual assault nurse examiners. Retrieved from https://www.forensicnurses.org/page/AboutSANE

International Society for Traumatic Stress Studies. (n.d.). Mission and strategic plan. Retrieved from https://www.istss.org/about-istss/strategic-plan.aspx

International Society of Psychiatric-Mental Health Nurses. (2018). About ISPN. Retrieved from http://www.ispn-psych.org/about-ispn

Krebs, C., Lindquist, C., Berzofsky, M., Shook-Sa, B., & Peterson, K. (2016). Campus climate survey validation study: Final technical report. Bureau of Justice Statistics and RTI International. Retrieved from https://www.bjs.gov/content/pub/pdf/ccsvsftr.pdf

Meyer, I. H. (2003). Prejudice, social stress, and mental health in lesbian, gay, and bisexual populations: Conceptual issues and research evidence. *Psychological Bulletin, 129*(5), 674–697. doi:10.1037/0033-2909.129.5.674

National Child Traumatic Stress Network. (n.d.). Who we are. Retrieved from https://www.nctsn.org/about-us/history-of-the-nctsn

National Child Traumatic Stress Network, Child Sexual Abuse Collaborative Group. (2014). *LGBTQ youth and sexual abuse: Information for mental health professionals.* Retrieved from https://www.nctsn.org/sites/default/files/resources//lgbtq_youth_sexual_abuse_professionals.pdf

National LGBT Health Education Center. (2018). What we offer. Retrieved from https://www.lgbthealtheducation.org/about-us/lgbt-health-education/

National Trauma Institute. (n.d.). About. Retrieved from https://ntrr-nti.org/about

National Trauma Institute. (2018). Mission. Retrieved from https://www.nattrauma.org/who-we-are/mission/

Regan, K. (2010). Trauma informed care on an inpatient pediatric psychiatric unit and the emergence of ethical dilemmas as nurses evolved their practice. *Issues in Mental Health Nursing, 31*(3), 216–222. doi:10.3109/0161284090331584

Society for the Advancement of Disaster Nursing. (2018). About. Retrieved from https://disasternursing.org/about/

Substance Abuse and Mental Health Administration. (n.d.). About us. Retrieved from https://www.samhsa.gov/about-us

Substance Abuse and Mental Health Services Administration. (2014). *SAMHSA's concept of trauma and guidance for a trauma-informed approach.* HHS Publication No. SMA 14-4884. Rockville, MD: Author.

US Department of Education. (2018). The Family Educational Rights and Privacy Act (FERPA). Retrieved from https://www2.ed.gov/policy/gen/guid/fpco/ferpa/index.html

US Department of Education, Office of Civil Rights. (2015). *Title IX resource guide.* Retrieved from https://www2.ed.gov/about/offices/list/ocr/docs/dcl-title-ix-coordinators-guide-201504.pdf

US Department of Health and Human Services. (2013). Summary of the HIPAA Privacy Rule. Retrieved from https://www.hhs.gov/hipaa/for-professionals/privacy/laws-regulations/index.html

US Department of Veterans Affairs. (2017). About PTSDpubs. Retrieved from https://www.ptsd.va.gov/PTSDpubs/index.asp

US Department of Veterans Affairs. (2018). PTSD: National Center for PTSD. Retrieved from https://www.ptsd.va.gov/

White House Task Force to Protect Students From Sexual Assault. (2017). *The second report of the White House Task Force to Protect Students From Sexual Assault.* Retrieved from http://www.changingourcampus.org/resources/not-alone/Second-Report-VAW-Event-TF-Report.PDF

LEARNING OBJECTIVES

At the end of this chapter, you will be able to:

- Appraise Florence Nightingale's approach to nursing as a practice profession and her creed to place our patients' needs first.
- Explain the interprofessional collaborations that may organically evolve in the care of patients who have experienced traumatic events.
- Deconstruct the trends surrounding trauma, nursing, and culture.
- Elaborate on personal, professional, and societal mechanisms to prevent and mitigate adverse childhood experiences (ACEs).
- Predict how efforts to prevent and mitigate ACEs will cascade into impacting intergenerational trauma.

CONCLUSIONS AND FUTURE DIRECTIONS 8

PURPOSE OF THE CHAPTER

We close this book by discussing current patterns and extending these into the future. Cumulative trends surrounding care are cited and described. Looking back on our historical iconic figure, Florence Nightingale, we gain glimpses into what must have been nursing care amidst patient trauma from war as well as nurses' secondary trauma. We look at the professional team members who contribute to our collaborative efforts in a trauma context. Evidence-based ways to interrupt the inter-generational cycles of adverse childhood experiences (ACEs) and forecasting future efforts are discussed. Last, we hypothesize where conversations about healing from trauma may take us—our hope is for a kinder, more compassionate sense of community, both at the micro and the macro levels.

LESSONS FROM FLORENCE NIGHTINGALE AND THE INTERPROFESSIONAL TEAM

From caricature to icon, Florence Nightingale was something in between. Criticized for her emphasis on the character of those recruited into nursing rather than education (Nelson & Rafferty, 2010), perhaps Nightingale's emphasis on character fits into our thesis about comfort being paramount to trauma-informed care (TIC). Looking back upon her role in caring for soldiers during the Crimean War, her environments must have been trauma-ridden. We can imagine the accounts of the horrors of war, the primitive medicine used in administering to the soldiers, and the nurses themselves, who surely must have been affected by such conditions.

Yet Nightingale concentrated on boundaries and purpose and the "doing" of nursing: putting the alleviation of patient suffering first. She is clear about nurses in the endnotes of *Notes on Nursing* (1859/2009) in discussing what nurses view as their "business"—tasks such as scouring floors that could be done by others:

> the good of their sick first, and second only in consideration what it was their "place" to do—and that women who wait for the housemaid to do this, or for the charwoman to do that, when their patients are suffering, have not the making of a nurse in them. (Chapter 1, Endnote No. 5)

What is our place today? Nurses placing the good of our patients first has carried us through the years and contributed to our selfless personas. But isn't there a balance needed as demonstrated by secondary trauma, compassion fatigue, second-victim trauma, and workplace violence? Haven't we reached a tipping point as a profession in which we must see that our rights are intricately intertwined with the safety and well-being of those we care for? Can't we be of noble and self-sacrificing character and still recognize that we are vulnerable to trauma?

We cannot do this alone. Individuals—wherever they are on the spectrum of care (promotion, prevention, or treatment)—need informed providers across disciplines. Depending upon the outcome of the trauma, professionals who are needed in a team-based care plan include:

- The individual who has experienced trauma

- Nurses (generalists and advanced practice)

- Physicians (generalists and multiple specialties, including psychiatrists)

- Physician assistants

- Social workers

- Psychologists and other mental health counselors

- Family life educators

- Certified nursing assistants

- Physical, occupational, and speech therapists

- Case managers

- Pharmacists

- First responders (for example, police officers, paramedics, emergency medical technicians, and firefighters)

- Volunteers (for example, court-appointed special advocates)

The time of professionals operating in silos is in the past. However, when thinking of those who have endured trauma, interprofessional cooperation and collaboration translates into continuity of care, communication via medical notes and electronic health records, and concentrated efforts to clarify needs born from trauma. Our healthcare system is often unfriendly to this model, which makes our efforts more difficult at times, but necessary. Karen asked her graduate students to describe nursing in contrast to other disciplines: "What is it that nurses do?" After a bit of discussion, the group seemed to arrive at this metaphor: "Nurses sew up the care for the patient. We fill in the gaps, ensure continuity, advocate for the patient, and communicate with everyone so that the treatment plan is solid." What an important role, and one that becomes even more vital when the patient has endured a traumatic event.

TRENDS IN TRAUMA-INFORMED (NURSING) CARE

Throughout this book, we've covered topics supported by the seminal, current, and best evidence. Here we cover some significant trends we've seen emerge as we have discussed various pockets of literature.

TRAUMA-INFORMED CARE IS BECOMING PART OF OUR DAILY LEXICON (THIS IS DISTINCT FROM CONVERSATIONS ABOUT TRAUMA/TRAUMA THEORY).

Originally published in 1962, Kuhn's *The Structure of Scientific Revolutions* (2012) described paradigm shifts, those ingrained patterns of thinking that are periodically displaced as new information takes hold in scientific thought. We believe this shift has already started and is becoming stronger. The impetus to this, in our opinion, is that psychological trauma is, sadly, so pervasive in today's world. While the reasons behind this remain complex and beyond the mission of this book, they nonetheless exist. In the postmodern world, language —the words we use—not only describes reality but also creates a new reality by its use. Such is the case with trauma. We have created a new reality that takes the secrets and stigma that often accompany trauma and moves them into our global culture and communities.

The good news is that nurses now know how important it is to recognize trauma, resilience, and posttraumatic growth so that comfort to self, patients, and community is based on current evidence. This openness brings us to our second trend: those in society who are influenced by trauma.

TRAUMA AFFECTS DIFFERENT SOCIAL UNITS, AND THE WORLD, AND THIS IS PART OF OUR CULTURE.

What once was considered an individual psychological phenomenon, we now recognize that social units, such as communities, may have experienced trauma as a collective. In the same way, healing may occur as communal events and projects. We have, then, become a trauma culture (Kaplan, 2005) post-9/11 that speaks to how we interpret and are influenced by communal traumatic stress. In the following passage, Kaplan (2005) describes New York City only four years after the attack on September 11, 2001, and how difficult it was for the "people to move on":

> to "working through," the stage of accepting what has happened, mourning the many kinds of loss, and providing—not closure or healing (the wound to New York will remain forever)—but a fitting witness, a fitting way to memorialize the catastrophe. (p. 136)

Kaplan (2005) describes how the people of New York and the US, collectively, experienced significant trauma. We see similarities between this description and the individual processes used after experiencing trauma: remaining with an event, remembering, loss, mourning, and acceptance.

TRAUMA AFFECTS EVERYONE, BUT SOME GROUPS ARE MORE VULNERABLE THAN OTHERS.

Through scientific publications that disseminate research findings to organizations such as the National Child Traumatic Stress Network, we understand that certain groups in society are more likely to be victims and survivors of trauma than others, including females, older adults, veterans, racial and ethnic minorities, those in the healthcare system, and those affected by socioeconomic disadvantages, social determinants of health, and gender orientation and sexual preferences. We see nurses as a vulnerable group, as asserted in this book. Due to the nature of our profession and the places in which we offer care, we are exposed to trauma almost daily.

As healthcare providers, thought leaders from the Institute for Healthcare Improvement (Berwick, Nolan, & Whittington, 2008) forwarded a "triple aim" for healthcare. One of these aims was the provision of quality services. Nurses, by understanding certain patients' vulnerabilities—and their own—can support equity in providing care and further advocate when necessary for such equity.

TRAUMA CONVERSATIONS NOW INCLUDE NURSES AS VICTIMS AND SURVIVORS OF TRAUMATIC EVENTS.

Historically, nurses have been identified as energy givers, on the sending end of services. This has cost us; many nurses have fallen into despair and exhaustion over the unrelenting feelings of empathy and compassion. Additionally, many of us have endured sexual harassment, workplace violence, incivility, unsafe staffing, and organizations that have left us voiceless.

Nurses have rallied together through policy efforts and organizations, such as the American Nurses Association and the American Academy of Nursing, to promote the good of the whole through safe staffing legislature, diversity initiatives, workplace violence awareness, and healthcare environments that acknowledge the presence of trauma. As this book's contents attest, we have much work to do so that others understand our value and vulnerabilities.

PERHAPS AS A RESULT OF THE TRENDS, ONE FINAL PATTERN APPEARS: EMPHASIS ON PREVENTION.

Awareness, the common experience of trauma, and trauma becoming mainstream allow us to expend energies in preventing or being ready for traumatic events to occur (for example, disaster preparedness and avoiding retraumatization). Evidence of these preventive efforts are Mental Health First Aid and Psychological First Aid (see Chapter 6). We discuss this as we move forward as a society and discuss states' efforts in preventing and mitigating the occurrences of ACEs.

TRAUMA-INFORMED REFLECTION

Select one or two of the five trends listed in this chapter (TIC is becoming part of our healing art and science; trauma affects different social units but is part of our culture; although no one is immune to trauma, vulnerable groups exist in society; nurses are now considered victims and survivors of trauma; and the emphasis on preventing trauma is growing). Discuss how you, as a person, may situate yourself into these trends. What goals can you formulate as you think about the future?

MOVING FORWARD AS A SOCIETY TO PROTECT FUTURE GENERATIONS

Throughout this book, and especially in Chapter 2, we discussed the types of trauma that individuals and nurses face. We positioned ACEs as one source of potential trauma in society. In an updated ACE study, Merrick, Ford, Ports, and Guinn (2018) found that in a sample of 214,157 individuals, 61.5% had experienced at least one ACE compared with 26% (Felitti et al., 1998), and 24.6% had experienced three or more ACEs compared with 9.5% (Felitti et al., 1998). The researchers also found groups that were more likely to have experienced adverse events: those who identified as black, Hispanic, or multiracial; those with less than a high school education; those earning less than $15,000 per year; those who were unemployed or unable to work; and those who were gay/lesbian or bisexual (Merrick et al., 2018). The most common ACEs reported were emotional abuse (34.4% compared with 11% [Felitti et al., 1998]), parental separation or divorce (27.6% compared with 23% [Felitti et al., 1998]), and finally, household substance abuse (27.5% compared with 27% [Felitti et al., 1998; Merrick et al., 2018).

As concerning as these findings are, it's important for us to emphasize that people are taking notice and actively engaged in interventions to prevent and mitigate the effects of early life trauma. Through these efforts, we hope to stop intergenerational trauma from proliferating and improve health across the life span. Specifically, in a report published by the National Conference of State Legislatures (Bellazaire, 2018), strategies in several states include building resilience through state-funded programs that include facilitating positive parenting skills through home visitation and supporting access to quality early childhood education. One of the strongest evidence-based programs is the Nurse-Family Partnership (2018), with outcomes supported by randomized control trials. The Nurse-Family Partnership aims to reach vulnerable mothers and babies to positively impact family health in 42 states, the Virgin Islands, and five tribal communities.

In addition to building resilience, a second area that has been targeted by states is an effort to decrease parental stress (Bellazaire, 2018). Financial hardship is one source of parental stress, and we know that young parents are especially vulnerable. Two concerning facts: 3.4 million children live with young parents, ages 18 to 24 years; and 37% of these children live in poverty—sometimes extreme poverty (69% live in families with incomes less than 200% of the federal poverty level). The median family income for these young parents is $23,000 per year (Annie E. Casey Foundation, 2018). Yet these parents are eager for accurate, quality knowledge about their children's growth and development. Many gaps exist in reaching parents with the information they need, despite our knowledge that such information impacts parenting behaviors (Bartlett, Guzman, & Ramos-Olazagasti, 2018). Several states have made efforts to reduce economic barriers by earned income tax credits, paying more than the minimum wage to workers, paid sick leave, and affordable housing (Bellazaire, 2018).

A third area that states are targeting is increasing screening and treatment related to mental and physical health needs (Bellazaire, 2018). In Chapter 3, we discuss how children, adolescents, and adults who have experienced ACEs are at risk for various difficulties in life, from emotional, mental, and behavioral disorders, including suicide, to aggression and poor job performance. With 27.5% of individuals reporting household substance abuse (Merrick et al., 2018), the third most prevalent ACE, one can quickly grasp the implications of the US's opioid crisis and the effect on children raised in these households. States are increasing efforts and broadening interventions to include children with parents struggling with substance use dependencies. For example, in Indiana, Senate Bill 446, passed in 2017 (residential substance abuse treatment), established a pilot program for new mothers and pregnant women with opioid addictions to receive residential care facility and home visitation services following discharge.

Sadly, evidence supports that harsh physical discipline (abuse) is perpetrated across generations; however, this can be decreased with positive relationships with parents, especially having a close relationship with a father (Herrenkohl, Klika, Brown, Herrenkohl, & Leeb, 2013). Further evidence of the significant impact that can be gained as a result of caring relationships was found by Thornberry et al. (2013). Safe, stable, and nurturing relationships (SSNRs) were found to act as direct protective factors, reducing risk of perpetuation of maltreatment (Thornberry et al., 2013). Thus, one conclusion is that while the risk exists for individuals who have been maltreated to become perpetrators, the presence of SSNRs has the potential to break this cycle. We hope that as you have read the preceding information, you stopped and contemplated how instrumental professional nurses are, and can continue to be, in these efforts. For every trauma we can prevent or encourage healing from, we are also impacting generations to come and contributing to the betterment of society.

TRAUMA-INFORMED REFLECTION

As a beginning generalist in nursing, what aspects of your practice have been impacted by reading this book? What three areas, as you progress in school and your career, have changed because of this information? In what domain have they changed: knowledge, affect/attitude, or tasks/skills?

We have one final story to share. (See "Camila's Story.") It's about a student nurse, a survivor, who decided to heal herself, and in the process, evolved into a professional who helps patients overcome trauma.

CAMILA'S STORY

At 18 years old, Camila felt different from other people—older in spirit and soul. It seemed as if she'd been an adult most of her life. Growing up in a household where the goal was to pay the bills and "put food on the table" did not leave much time for her single mom to spend with her four brothers and herself. She often would see her mom get high and not come home at night. The second eldest child and being the only girl, she was the one upon whom her mother depended for taking care of the younger kids, cooking, and keeping things at home in order. At times, it was a choice between feeding her siblings or herself, so she'd go hungry occasionally. She and her brothers had even been placed in foster care for two weeks when she was 12. She'd never forget being moved into a strange home, separated from her brothers. The people were nice enough, but it felt like a military camp—more rules than she could keep track of. She'd never been able to shake the fear she felt during those 15 days, wondering where her brothers were, how long she would have to live there, what was happening to her belongings, and why her mother didn't come for her. She remembers the caseworker talking to the foster mom about removing the children due to severe neglect and how neither "the father" nor any relatives could be located.

Now, finally, it was her turn, and she was putting all this pain behind her. It was finally her time to explore life.

She'd rented a small apartment with two other girls and enrolled in a two-year nursing degree program offered by her community college. She'd even been fortunate enough to earn some scholarship money and take out a loan to pay for the rent, tuition, and books. Yet, on her first day, looking at the other students, she didn't feel good enough to be there. She wondered whether any of them had ever been placed in foster care. But she was determined to be the top student in class. After all, hard work was something she knew very well.

One of her roommates and friend, Elise, noticed Camila worked night and day and had taken a part-time job to help her brothers. Camila had a 4.0 grade point average—straight A's. She'd also noticed Camila was dating several guys and wearing more makeup and revealing clothing, and experimenting with alcohol. One guy in particular, David, was pulling Camila in ways that made Elise uneasy, including buying her hard liquor. When she asked Camila about him, Camila said, "I think he's the first person who's ever really loved me."

Camila maintained her GPA until the beginning of her second year. She and David had been together for six months, and she'd gotten drunk more and more frequently since dating him. She suspected he was seeing other people and grew increasingly obsessed with him, begging him to commit to her. One night, she became so intoxicated that she couldn't remember what had happened to her, only that when she woke, she was unclothed from the waist down, and there were several men in the next room of David's apartment.

She quickly dressed, locked herself in the bedroom, and walked home as soon as David assured her all the others had left. At first, he was angry when she wouldn't come out, but then later, he soothed her and said that only the two of them had been intimate. "I'd never let another guy touch you!" Later that day, she skipped class, and when Elise arrived at the apartment, Camila told her what had happened. They talked for hours. Camila began to think about all she'd been though in her life. She hated what she'd become, but her need to feel loved and recognized had motivated her to make choices that were unhealthy. Her psychiatric-mental health nursing class had talked about trauma; she fit several of the characteristics of a woman whose child-hood had been marked by emotional and physical neglect. There had been no adult to make her feel valued, loved, nurtured, cared for. In turn, she had neglected herself. Perhaps subconsciously, she had been the overachiever, seeking validation from external rewards—anything to make her feel worthy. She'd clung to David, who at first made her feel so special.

Elise told her about a community counseling center with a sliding scale and helped Camila set up an appointment. She also had a physical and was tested for sexually transmitted diseases. Through the next months, Camila stopped drinking, and after attending a few Alcoholics Anonymous meet-ings, believed she was not dependent. Although in some ways she'd become addicted to David, she broke up with him and began to understand what a balance in life was. She forced herself to have downtime when she wasn't working and began taking yoga classes and meditating. She saw her brothers often but was able to put her needs at least in equal measure to theirs. She rarely saw her mother, who was the subject of many therapy sessions. Her therapist helped her process the neglect and the trauma of being placed in foster care. She mourned the loss of a childhood that would have allowed her to just be a child. She grieved for what should have been basic parenting in her life and processed the anger at what could have been. And she learned the value of positive relationships, such as she had with Elise. She learned about self-compassion and forgiveness and valued the compassion shown by her therapist. She accepted that, although she had been through so much during her youth, she had also shown resiliency and strength. She began to appreciate how she had shown care and love toward her brothers, despite the pain she had endured.

Camila graduated with her associate's degree and began practicing in a general medical-surgical unit. After a year, she decided to return to school for her bachelor's degree through an online program. From there, she secured a position as a staff nurse on a psychiatric inpatient unit and finished her degree. After working with patients and knowing she had more to offer, she completed her education as an advanced practice psychiatric-mental health nurse practitioner. Employed by a general hospital, she balances a small outpatient practice and consult-liaison work where she advises on inpatient hospitalized patients' needs. She counsels many patients who have experienced trauma and understands firsthand what healing and recovery are about.

CLOSING THOUGHTS

This conversation—our narratives with yours—is the beginning of our movement forward. Through these pages, you've become sensitive to this whole "thing" we call trauma. You now have the knowledge, possess attitudes and beliefs, and grasp the skills and resources to move forward in a trauma-informed way. We are being presented with a wonderful opportunity: to make a positive difference in the world. At times, it may be easier for us to become hardened by life, to choose not to empathize with the pain of others, to become a person enthralled with personal satisfaction and in-the-moment pleasures, and to deny our own personal trauma secrets and avoid the secrets of others. Miller (2007) refers to "illegitimate hatred" (p. 115), extending a thesis that ideologies and national/tribal hatreds are connected to childhood trauma and injuries. Yet such illegitimate hatred never disappears or can be appeased as innocent people are scapegoated (Miller, 2007, p. 115). Only when there is recognition—an acknowledgment of the trauma and an understanding of those responsible—can illegitimate hatred dissipate and recovery occur.

We believe that nurses are offered a different path to take—one of self-awareness, courage, and compassion. Nursing is all-encompassing. It becomes more than what you do; it's who you are. Although this book is not one of morality, we believe that taking a path toward healing from trauma is the right path. For those of us who are nurses, this path becomes blurred between the personal and the professional. We see this not as an impediment but an enormous opportunity to grow as a person. In a world of divisiveness and tribal separations, being a trauma-informed caregiver is a vehicle of healing in multiple ways.

Our wish for you is to experience life with an abundance of happiness, satisfaction, courage, and compassion, undiminished by the negative effects of stress and trauma. Second, we hope that you extend to yourself, to your friends and family, and to individuals in need of nursing care and comfort, interactions characterized by kindness that apply your trauma-informed knowledge. And last, we hope that you share what you have learned with others. They're all waiting for our help.

HIGHLIGHTS OF CHAPTER CONTENT

- Florence Nightingale emphasized that nursing care is to be directed by patient needs rather than by professional boundaries.
- Teams of professionals that span disciplines and roles provide continuity in trauma-informed care.
- Trends in trauma-informed nursing care include incorporating this subject into our daily lexicon, recognizing trauma as a presence in social units and our culture, understanding vulnerable groups, acknowledging that nurses are survivors of traumatic events, and focusing on trauma prevention.
- Strategic forces, including state legislatures and healthcare partnerships, are diligently working to prevent and mitigate early life trauma; to this end, intergenerational trauma may be lessened.

REFERENCES

Annie E. Casey Foundation. (2018). *Opening doors for young parents*. Baltimore, MD: Author. Retrieved from https://www.aecf.org/m/resourcedoc/aecf-openingdoorsforyoungparents-2018.pdf

Bartlett, J. D., Guzman, L., & Ramos-Olazagasti, M. A. (2018). *Knowledge among first-time parents of young children* [Research brief]. Retrieved from https://www.childtrends.org/wp-content/uploads/2018/07/ParentingKnowledge_ChildTrends_July2018.pdf

Bellazaire, A. (2018). *Preventing and mitigating the effects of adverse childhood experiences*. National Conference of State Legislatures. Retrieved from http://www.ncsl.org/Portals/1/HTML_LargeReports/ACEs_2018_32691.pdf

Berwick, D. M., Nolan, T. W., & Whittington, J. (2008). The triple aim: Care, health, and cost. *Health Affairs, 27*(3), 759–769.

Felitti, V. J., Anda, R. F., Nordenberg, D., Williamson, D. F., Spitz, A. M., Edwards, V., . . . Marks, J. S. (1998). Relationship of childhood abuse and household dysfunction to many of the leading causes of death in adults: The Adverse Childhood Experiences (ACE) study. *American Journal of Preventive Medicine, 14*(4), 245–258.

Herrenkohl, T. I., Klika, J. B., Brown, E. C., Herrenkohl, R. C., & Leeb, R. T. (2013). Tests of mitigating effects of caring and supportive relationships in the study of abusive disciplining over two generations. *Journal of Adolescent Health, 53*, S18–S24. doi:http://dx.doi.org/10.1016/j.jadohealth.2013.04.009

Kaplan, E. A. (2005). *Trauma culture: The politics of terror and loss in the media and literature*. New Brunswick, New Jersey: Rutgers University Press.

Kuhn, T. (2012). *The structure of scientific revolutions*. Chicago, IL: University of Chicago Press.

Merrick, M. T., Ford, D. C., Ports, K. A., & Guinn, A. S. (2018). Prevalence of adverse childhood experiences from the 2011–2014 behavioral risk factor surveillance system in 23 states. *JAMA Pediatrics, 172*(11), 1038–1044. doi:10.1001/jamapediatrics.2018.2537

Miller, A. (2007). *The drama of the gifted child: The search for the true self*. New York, NY: Basic Books.

Nelson, S., & Rafferty, A. M. (2010). *Notes on Nightingale: The influence and legacy of a nursing icon*. Ithaca, NY: Cornell University Press.

Nightingale, F. (1859/2009). *Notes on nursing*. New York, NY: Fall River Press.

Nurse-Family Partnership. (2018). About us. Retrieved from https://www.nursefamilypartnership.org/about/

Thornberry, T. P., Henry, K. L., Smith, C. A., Ireland, T. O., Greenman, S. J., & Lee, R. D. (2013). Breaking the cycle of maltreatment: The role of safe, stable, and nurturing relationships. *Journal of Adolescent Health, 53*, S25–S31. doi:http://dx.doi.org/10.1016/j.jadohealth.2013.04.019

GLOSSARY

Acute trauma: Trauma occurring as a single event or for a limited time. See also chronic trauma; complex trauma; developmental trauma; historical trauma; secondary trauma; second-victim trauma; treatment trauma.

Adherence: The degree to which an individual/patient follows a medication regimen, plan of treatment, and other medical instructions. Past trauma may influence adherence.

Adverse childhood experiences (ACEs): Stressful and potentially traumatic experiences in childhood categorized as abuse, household challenges, and neglect; higher ACE scores are associated with decreased mortality and increased morbidity.

Child maltreatment: Abuse and neglect that children and youth experience.

Chronic trauma: Trauma that is sustained, repeated, and prolonged. See also acute trauma, complex trauma; developmental trauma; historical trauma; secondary trauma; second-victim trauma; treatment trauma.

Compassion: A choice made by caregivers to demonstrate empathy, kindness, concern, and a willingness to help toward self (self-compassion), patients (compassion and compassion satisfaction), and team members (team compassion).

Compassion fatigue: Expenditure of compassion due to psychological caring efforts that is in excess of emotional resources; psychological recovery is needed to be fully present to patients. See also secondary traumatic stress (STS).

Complex trauma (interpersonal trauma): Trauma inflicted by caregivers and others trusted to provide for the physical and emotional needs of the child. See also acute trauma, chronic trauma; developmental trauma; historical trauma; secondary trauma; second-victim trauma; treatment trauma.

Developmental trauma: Trauma that negatively impacts the developmental trajectory of children and youth. See also acute trauma, chronic trauma; complex trauma; historical trauma ; secondary trauma; second-victim trauma; treatment trauma.

Duck Syndrome: Young adults who appear to be high functioning but who are actually struggling with the pressures and expectations of life.

Family Educational Rights and Privacy Act (FERPA): This law protects students' educational records and applies to organizations that receive funds from the Department of Education; rights are transferred from the parents to the student at 18 years.

Health Insurance Portability and Accountability Act (HIPAA): This federal law pertains to an individual's protected health information and the penalties for violations of the patient's privacy.

Historical trauma (intergenerational trauma): Trauma passed down to future generations so that the offspring are vulnerable to the original trauma. See also acute trauma, chronic trauma; complex trauma; developmental trauma; second-victim trauma; secondary trauma; treatment trauma.

Horizontal and lateral violence (incivility in nursing): Attitudes, actions, or behaviors, such as bullying and other forms of aggression, from one dominant individual or group to a less powerful individual or group that may result in trauma.

Intrusion symptoms: A diagnostic criterion for posttraumatic stress disorder, these symptoms are involuntary and distressing, taking the form of memories, dreams, flashbacks, and physiological reactions. See also posttraumatic stress disorder; posttraumatic stress symptoms.

Journaling (narrative discourse): A narrative surrounding trauma or a traumatic event with the goal of revealing a new coherence.

Leininger, Madeleine: See theory of culture care diversity and universality.

Mantram meditation: Softly repeating affirming, short, existing phrases while meditating.

Mental Health First Aid: A community-based training program designed to promote recovery and resiliency for those experiencing mental health illnesses. See also Psychological First Aid.

Mindfulness: Paying attention with an open mind, in the present moment, and withholding judgment.

Neglect: Failure of caregivers to meet the basic physical and emotional needs of the child, youth, adult, or older adult. Neglect is considered to be traumatic to the individual.

Neurobiology of trauma: Physiologic changes in the brain that result from exposure to trauma.

NotAlone: Originating from the White House Task Force to Protect Students from Sexual Assault in 2014, NotAlone was established to raise awareness of sexual assault, communicate to survivors that they are not alone, and let them know that resources are available in colleges and universities to assist survivors. See also Title IX of the Education Amendments of 1972.

Peplau, Hildegard: See Theory of interpersonal relations.

Poly-victimization: Children and youth who experience multiple types of trauma.

Posttraumatic growth: Improvement in psychological functioning after experiencing trauma; coming through a difficult time with more (insight, relationships, and personal philosophy) than the person possessed prior to the event.

Posttraumatic stress disorder (PTSD): A diagnostic term described by criteria in the *Diagnostic and Statistical Manual of Mental Disorders,* Fifth Edition (DSM-5) for adults, adolescents, and children.

Posttraumatic stress symptoms (PTSS): Components, signs, and symptoms used to diagnose posttraumatic stress disorder. One example is cognitive deficits.

Psychological First Aid: A training program for first responders and other disaster workers designed to reduce the impact of trauma post-disaster and post-terrorist events. See also Mental Health First Aid.

Resilience: Positive adaption following a potentially traumatic event that can manifest as a trait, a process, a defense mechanism, or an outcome.

Retraumatization: Going back into a trauma state, triggered by an event.

Sanctuary Model: A model of trauma-informed care delivery that acknowledges the role of trauma on those served by organizations, on those in serving roles, and on the organizational culture itself.

SANE designation: A certification that designates a nurse has taken training to become a Sexual Assault Nurse Examiner (SANE) to deliver comprehensive and compassionate care to individuals who have experienced sexual assault.

Secondary trauma (indirect trauma/vicarious trauma): The nurse, through witnessing or living through others' trauma, may begin to experience secondary posttraumatic stress symptoms. In these instances, nurses are not experiencing firsthand trauma but experiencing the symptoms related to having gone through such stress. See also acute trauma; chronic trauma; complex trauma; developmental trauma; historical trauma; second-victim trauma; treatment trauma.

Secondary traumatic stress (STS): Stress experienced by the healthcare worker as a result of caring for traumatized individuals.

Second-victim trauma: The trauma that the nurse may experience as a result of a medical error or adverse event. See also acute trauma; chronic trauma; complex trauma; developmental trauma; historical trauma; secondary trauma; treatment trauma.

Sexual orientation and gender identity: Individuals' identities are seen along continuums signifying biological sex, gender identity, gender expression, and sexual orientation.

Social support: Tangible and intangible resources that family and friends offer to act as buffers to and mitigate stress and trauma. Social support contributes to feelings of interpersonal connectedness.

Theory of culture care diversity and universality (Madeleine Leininger): A nursing theory that describes both cultural care universality, which acknowledges humanity's common, similar, and uniform meanings, and culture care diversity, which are culturally derived meanings and values.

Theory of interpersonal relations (Hildegard Peplau): A nursing theory that centers nursing care on the nurse-patient relationship and the essential need for this relationship; nurses observe both themselves and the patients as interactions occur.

Theory of transpersonal caring/Caring Science (Jean Watson): A complex theory related to experiencing being a human in new and different ways, emphasizing lovingkindness to self and others. Caritas or loving care is a central concept to this theory.

Three E's of trauma: The three E's—Event, Experience, and Effects—examine how individuals react to, process, and make sense of trauma.

Title IX of the Education Amendments of 1972 (Title IX): This federal law protects students, employees, and applicants for admission and employment from all forms of sex discrimination, including those nonconforming to stereotypical notions of gender.

Toxic stress: Exposure to stress that is intense, prolonged, and severe, resulting in various negative outcomes such as dysregulation and maladaptive coping.

Trauma-informed (nursing) care (TIC): An approach to nursing care that incorporates the six guiding principles of TIC: 1) safety; 2) trustworthiness and transparency; 3) peer support and mutual self-help; 4) collaboration and mutuality; 5) empowerment, voice, and choice; and 6) cultural, historical, and gender issues.

Trauma-informed schools (K-12): Schools from kindergarten to high school are changing their habits, customs, and culture to become trauma-informed so that students who have experienced trauma may feel safe and be in an environment conducive to learning.

Trauma surrounding disasters: Although disasters vary in scope and fluidity, nurses may be involved as first responders, putting them at risk for direct and secondary trauma. See also Psychological First Aid; secondary trauma.

Trauma triggers: A stimulus, usually perceived through the senses, that creates a link to a previous traumatic experience.

Treatment trauma (system-induced trauma): The diagnosis (sudden/ catastrophic) or healthcare treatment that causes the individual to experience trauma/traumatic stress.

Watson, Jean: See theory of transpersonal caring/Caring Science.

Ways of knowing: Building on the four ways of knowing identified by Carper, which include empirical, esthetic, ethical, and personal self. Chinn and Kramer have added a fifth way: emancipatory knowing.

Workplace violence: Verbal, written, or physical abuse/assault from patients and visitors directed toward nurses. Workplace violence also includes nurse-to-nurse horizontal violence (incivility). See also horizontal and lateral violence.

INDEX

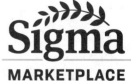

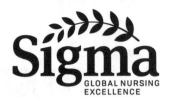
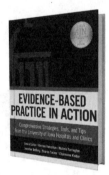
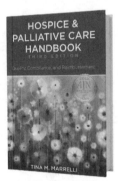
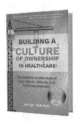
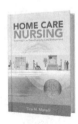
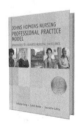
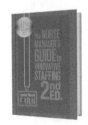